Rebuild & Thrive

Vol. 3

CHAIR YOGA BIBLE TO LOSE WEIGHT AND INCREASE FLEXIBILITY

DR. HAMRICK NELSON

Disclaimer

The exercises and information presented in this book are designed to promote health, stability, and well-being. However, it's important to remember that everyone's body is different, and what works well for one person may not be suitable for another. Before starting any new exercise program, especially if you have any pre-existing medical conditions or concerns, please consult with your doctor or healthcare provider to ensure these routines are safe for you.

While every effort has been made to ensure that the exercises are easy to follow and safe, your health and safety are our top priority. It's important to listen to your body—if you experience any discomfort or pain while performing any exercise, stop immediately and seek guidance from a healthcare professional. This book is intended to be a helpful guide, but it should not replace professional medical advice.

Dr. Hamrick Nelson and the team are committed to your well-being and encourage you to approach these exercises with care, patience, and an understanding of your body's needs.

The goal is to help you live a healthier, more active life, one step—or chair yoga—at a time.

Table of Contents

ABOUT THE AUTHOR

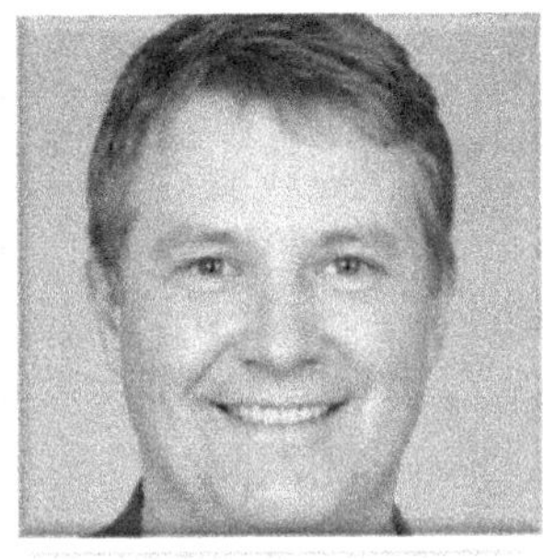

Dr. Hamrick Nelson is a leading voice in fitness and wellness, with a deep passion for helping individuals of all ages live healthier, more active lives. With over two decades of experience in the health and fitness industry, Dr. Nelson has dedicated his career to promoting accessible exercise routines for people at every stage of life. His approach is rooted in the belief that movement is for everyone, regardless of age or physical limitations.

While Dr. Nelson's work spans a wide range of fitness disciplines, he has a special focus on supporting seniors—particularly those over 60. Through his extensive research and hands-on experience, he understands the unique challenges faced by older adults, and he's made it his mission to help them maintain their independence, strength, and vitality. He combines practical knowledge with compassion, creating tailored fitness programs that prioritize safety and long-term health benefits.

Holding advanced degrees in physical therapy and exercise science, Dr. Nelson has worked with countless individuals to enhance their mobility, flexibility, and overall well-being. His books, workshops, and speaking engagements reflect his commitment to helping people of all ages—whether young or senior—stay fit, feel strong, and live life to the fullest.

His program offers an approachable, supportive path to better health, empowering older adults to continue thriving well into their golden years.

.

INTRODUCTION

This guide is more than just a collection of workouts; it's a path to a stronger, more flexible, and healthier you—right from the comfort of your chair. Whether you want to restore mobility, lose weight, or simply find an exercise regimen that works with your body's rhythm, you've come to the correct place.

My experiences as a health practitioner, as well as a narrative about Everard, inspired the inspiration for this book. Everard and I met by happenstance at one of my wellness classes several years ago. He was in his mid-sixties, had retired from engineering, and had spent his life doing manual labor and working long hours. Though once active, he was now dealing with weight gain, joint pain, and a gradual loss of flexibility. Everard's lifestyle had changed dramatically after he stopped working, and he found himself more limited to his home than he had anticipated.

Everard came to me hoping to restore his lost energy and reduce some weight, but he felt dissatisfied and defeated. With so many physical constraints, he couldn't simply start a high-intensity training routine or go to the gym like he used to. He also didn't consider himself to fit into the traditional definition of a fitness devotee. That's when I introduced him to chair yoga—specifically, a chair yoga practice meant to increase his metabolism, enhance his flexibility, and promote gradual weight loss. His reaction astonished me. Everard had always connected yoga with extreme flexibility and seemed afraid of doing it from a chair. But he trusted the process, and over several months, he set out on this journey to become a better version of himself.

When I first saw Everard settle into a seated mountain posture, I could tell he was uncomfortable. Not from the stretch itself, but from the mental challenge of sitting in a chair, performing yoga, and calling it "exercise." Within weeks, he noticed himself becoming stronger and more agile, and that mental barrier began to fade. Everard began to notice the results—not just on the scale, but in his everyday life. His energy level climbed, his posture improved, and the sense of defeat was gradually replaced with confidence. Everard's change sparked the idea for this book.

This path, like Everard's, can benefit you as well. Each chapter in this book is thoughtfully organized to walk you through every facet of chair yoga, including extensive instructions on form, breathing methods, and nutritional advice to supplement your practice. The exercises are intended to help you progress safely and methodically. And, much as I worked closely with Everard to adapt his approach, this book includes changes for every fitness level—whether you're just getting started or have been on a fitness journey for a while.

One of the major benefits of chair yoga is its accessibility. Traditional exercise might be difficult for people who have joint discomfort, restricted mobility or are searching for a low-impact alternative to stay active. Chair yoga makes training accessible to everyone, regardless of age or fitness level, and provides a unique combination of mild muscle growth, flexibility, and weight loss support.

Most significantly, chair yoga focuses on consistency over intensity. As Everard discovered, when you include little, consistent actions into your daily life, they begin to aggregate and produce obvious results. His original weight loss objectives were modest, but after months of consistent practice, he had exceeded his expectations. His mobility improved, his posture adjusted, and he even started doing breathing exercises, which helped him handle stress and sleep better. His progress was not quick, but it was consistent and, most importantly, sustainable.

In producing this guide, I concentrated on several basic themes that I've observed impact lives:

❖ ***Easy Weight Loss Techniques:*** Each exercise in this book has been carefully picked to help you burn calories efficiently while avoiding the strain associated with high-intensity activities. You don't need fancy equipment or pricey gym memberships; all you need is a chair, your body, and the determination to complete this adventure.

❖ ***Safe and Sustainable Mobility Improvements:*** One of the key goals of chair yoga is to help you regain your mobility of movement, not merely lose weight. Whether you're reaching for something on a high shelf, walking up stairs with ease, or simply feeling more solid on your feet, the exercises in this book will help you improve your balance, stability, and coordination.

❖ ***Mind-Body Connection:*** The breathing techniques and mindfulness activities described here seek to improve not just physical health but also mental well-being. Weight loss is not only a physical struggle but also a mental one. Everard explained that the mindful breathing techniques he acquired made him feel more grounded and less prone to stress eating, which he had suffered with for years. Similar approaches will help you tackle weight loss holistically.

❖ ***Motivation and Self-Tracking:*** Staying motivated during a fitness journey is typically one of the most difficult obstacles. This book is designed to help you set attainable goals and track your progress. I'll also tell the stories of others, such as Everard, who have altered their health through chair yoga. Remember that every modest accomplishment represents a step forward, and your success is unique to you.

Just as I saw Everard transform through his practice, I am convinced that with dedication and commitment, you will reap comparable results. The beauty of this journey is that it will be unique to each individual. Chair yoga, when combined with a balanced diet and a consistent program, has the potential to produce significant long-term results.

Imagine a future in which simple, daily activities give you more influence over your health and wellness. Imagine yourself feeling lighter, more mobile, and in tune with your body's rhythm. This book will guide you step by step in that path.

You don't need any prior yoga expertise, and you don't have to be in top form to begin. All you need is a chair, the will to attempt, and a commitment to your health. So let's prepare to begin this voyage together. The journey may not be easy, but with patience, persistence, and the correct tools, you can become a healthier, happier, and more mobile version of yourself.

Welcome to "Rebuild & Thrive Vol. 3". Let us begin.

CHAPTER 1: COMPREHENDING CHAIR YOGA AND LOSING WEIGHT

Chair Yoga's History

Chair yoga is a contemporary adaptation of traditional yoga designed to make it more accessible to older adults, people with restricted mobility, and people recovering from injuries. The spirit of yoga is retained, but the poses are modified to be done while sitting in a chair or with the chair supporting you. It is essential to look at both the historical context of yoga and the more recent developments that resulted in the creation of this modified form in order to fully understand the origins of chair yoga.

Ancient India is where yoga first appeared more than 5,000 years ago. It started as a philosophical and spiritual practice meant to unite the body, mind, and soul. Vedic texts, especially the Rigveda, which includes hymns and rituals conducted by Vedic priests, provide the first known descriptions of yoga. Over time, yoga developed into a more systematic practice, and by 500 BCE, it had been developed further in the Bhagavad Gita and the Upanishads, two of the most significant spiritual texts in Hindu philosophy.

In his ***"Yoga Sutras,"*** composed between 300 BCE and 500 CE, Patanjali categorized yoga into the eight-limbed Ashtanga style, emphasizing meditation, physical postures (asanas), breath control (pranayama), and moral principles. During this period, yoga was largely a spiritual practice aimed at attaining enlightenment, with little emphasis on physical poses.

With the advent of Hatha Yoga in the eleventh century, the physical aspect of yoga as we know it now initially gained prominence. Hatha Yoga established the foundation for many contemporary yoga styles, including chair yoga, and placed a strong emphasis on physical postures and breath control to prime the body for meditation.

As yoga spread outside of India in the nineteenth and twentieth centuries, it saw significant alterations. Yoga was brought to the West by Indian gurus such as Swami Vivekananda and Paramahansa Yogananda in the late 1800s and early 1900s. Although this was the beginning of a worldwide yoga movement, the emphasis remained mostly on the philosophical and spiritual elements rather than the physical poses that we now associate with yoga.

The physical advantages of yoga were well-known by the middle of the 20th century. Prominent instructors of yoga, such as B.K.S. Iyengar and T. Krishnamacharya played a significant part in popularizing yoga poses, or asanas, and opening up yoga to a larger audience. The physical exercises we see in yoga studios all over the world today are a direct result of their teachings. Iyengar specifically emphasized the use of chairs, belts, and blocks as props to help trainees achieve perfect alignment and prevent injuries.

It was in this setting that chair yoga first appeared. As yoga's popularity grew, instructors and practitioners realized that the practice needed to be modified to suit people who might find it difficult to perform standard yoga postures due to age, disability, or injury. By employing a chair as support, students could practice yoga without having to lie on their backs or perform difficult poses.

Although chair yoga's exact origins are uncertain, its development is closely linked to the late 20th-century emergence of adapted yoga. One kind of yoga designed especially for those with physical disabilities is called adaptive yoga. It makes yoga more accessible by modifying traditional poses to suit different skill levels.

Chair yoga's formalization is frequently attributed to yoga instructor and adaptive yoga pioneer Lakshmi Voelker. Voelker started working with clients who had mobility issues in the late

1980s, mostly elderly and disabled individuals. After seeing firsthand how difficult it was for many of her students to complete common yoga postures, she set out to find a way to make yoga more approachable for them.

Voelker developed a series of chair-based poses that could be done standing or sitting with the aid of a chair, drawing on her extensive knowledge of Hatha and Iyengar Yoga. She gave the novel method the name "Chair Yoga" and began instructing her students. She established the "Lakshmi Voelker Chair Yoga" certification program in 1987, formalizing her teachings. Since then, it has trained thousands of instructors all over the world.

Voelker's chair yoga classes quickly became well-liked, especially by the elderly and those with physical disabilities. Her approach emphasized traditional yoga concepts like alignment, awareness, and breath control while adapting the poses to make them safe and approachable for everyone. People who would not otherwise be able to participate in yoga were able to benefit from its many mental and physical advantages thanks to chair yoga.

The elderly, who often have movement difficulties that make regular yoga difficult, are particularly fond of chair yoga. Decreased strength, flexibility, and balance are associated with aging and are necessary for performing standing yoga poses.

For seniors who want to strengthen these areas without overtaxing their joints or running the danger of falling, chair yoga offers a mild, low-impact method.

Chair yoga has been shown to improve seniors' emotional health in addition to their physical health. Studies have demonstrated that yoga, particularly chair yoga, can help older adults feel less stressed, depressed, and anxious. Seniors experiencing the psychological impacts of aging, such as chronic pain or loss of independence, may benefit most from the practice's emphasis on mindfulness and relaxation.

For elders, chair yoga is a great way to foster social relationships. Group chair yoga classes reduce the loneliness and isolation that elderly people commonly feel by providing a welcoming environment in which participants can interact with others.

Additionally, chair yoga has gained popularity as a therapeutic method for individuals recovering from chronic diseases or accidents. Patients recuperating from hip or knee replacements, as well as those with multiple sclerosis or arthritis, are sometimes advised to do chair yoga by physical therapists and rehabilitation specialists. Because chair yoga is gentle, it's a safe and efficient way to regain mobility, strength, and flexibility without making existing issues worse.

People with disabilities can benefit from yoga in a more inclusive environment with chair yoga. Wheelchair users, people with neurological illnesses that limit their mobility, and people with various physical issues can all benefit from chair yoga. Everyone may perform modified versions of traditional yoga postures by using a chair as a prop, which provides the stability and support needed.

Nowadays, most people consider chair yoga to be a convenient and efficient kind of exercise. It is utilized in a variety of settings, such as business offices, rehabilitation clinics, and senior facilities. Anyone looking for a milder form of traditional yoga can practice chair yoga, but it's particularly common in health programs for the elderly, disabled, and those recovering from ailments.

People can now practice chair yoga from the comfort of their homes thanks to the availability of online yoga courses and instructional videos. Whether used for physical rehabilitation, stress relief, or overall health, chair yoga has emerged as a practical and versatile form of exercise that is becoming more and more well-liked.

The need for more accessible and inclusive yoga styles led to the development of chair yoga. Although it has been adapted to meet the needs of modern practitioners, especially those with restricted mobility, its roots are in the ancient yoga traditions. Chair yoga is a modern example of yoga's versatility and ability to help people of different ages and abilities.

Chair Yoga Styles

People who struggle with movement, balance, or performing exercises on the ground can benefit from chair yoga, which offers the benefits of traditional yoga but is more accessible. Elderly people, people recuperating from injuries, people with disabilities, and everyone else seeking a gentle, low-impact workout will find it particularly helpful. Through chair yoga, practitioners can improve their strength, flexibility, and balance without overtaxing their muscles or joints. Chair yoga comes in a variety of forms to accommodate varying demands and levels of fitness. The focus, level of intensity, and target audience set these chair yoga variations apart. Let's examine the most popular chair yoga styles and how different practitioners can benefit from them.

1. Yoga in a Seated Chair

The most fundamental kind of chair yoga is called "seated chair yoga," in which all of the poses are done while seated in a rigid chair. People who have limited mobility, are elderly or are recovering from ailments that prevent them from standing or balancing comfortably would benefit greatly from this type of chair yoga. In sitting chair yoga, the chair serves as a prop and a support system to help modify traditional yoga poses.

Seated Mountain Pose, Seated Forward Bend, Seated Cat-Cow, and Seated Spinal Twist are among the most popular poses in seated chair yoga. While maintaining the practitioner's chair-based stability, these poses enhance posture, flexibility, and core strength.

People who are unable to engage in regular standing exercises can still benefit from the mental and physical aspects of yoga thanks to seated chair yoga, which is one of its main advantages. People with arthritis or chronic pain can benefit greatly from it because it is easy on the joints and can be done practically anywhere, including in an office chair, a wheelchair, or a chair at home.

2. Supported Standing Chair Yoga

By employing the chair as support for standing poses, standing-supported chair yoga takes it a step further. This type of yoga allows the practitioner to perform poses with one or both hands resting on the chair or to hang onto it for balance while standing. For those who can stand and balance for a short while but need more help, standing-supported chair yoga is ideal.

Chair Warrior I, II, and III, Chair Tree Pose, and Chair Sun Salutation are all standing-supported chair yoga poses. While the chair's support offers stability and reduces the risk of falling, these standing poses improve leg strength, balance, and coordination. For those who spend a lot of time sitting down or have weak circulation, standing-supported chair yoga is perfect because it also enhances circulation, especially in the lower body.

This kind of chair yoga is perfect for building stamina and strength in a secure environment. It can be adjusted according to the practitioner's physical capabilities to accommodate varying degrees of fitness. People can progress to more challenging types and reduce their dependency on the chair for support as their balance improves.

3. Chair yoga for Flexibility and Mobility

Two crucial components of physical health, especially as people age, are mobility and flexibility. Improving the range of motion, especially in the joints, muscles, and connective tissues, is the goal of chair yoga for mobility and flexibility. For stiff people, who have joint issues, or want to become more flexible without running the risk of injury, this type of chair yoga is perfect.

Seated Forward Bends, Seated Leg Lifts, Chair Hip Stretches, and Seated Side Bends are chair yoga poses that increase flexibility and mobility. These exercises gently encourage joint mobility while lengthening and stretching muscles. For instance, while Seated Leg Lifts work the thighs and hip flexors, Seated Forward Bends stretch the hamstrings and lower back.

Frequent chair yoga for flexibility and mobility can help prevent injuries, lessen stiffness, and enhance general movement patterns. Because it helps to relax tense muscles and increase circulation, it is particularly beneficial for those who have arthritis or spend a lot of time sitting down.

4. Strength and Endurance Chair Yoga

Building strength is a crucial aspect of overall health, particularly for elderly people who may see a decline in muscle mass as they age. Chair yoga for strength and endurance is designed to help people build muscle and endurance, which enhances posture, balance, and everyday movements.

In chair yoga for strength, poses are often held for long periods to build endurance and engage muscles. Strengthening chair yoga exercises include Seated Squats, Chair Push-ups, and Seated Chair Tappers. These exercises provide a low-impact method of muscle building without the use of weights or resistance bands, and they focus on the legs, core, and upper body.

Chair yoga can help the elderly and those with mobility issues acquire independence, improve their balance and coordination, and reduce their risk of falling. People recuperating from injuries benefit greatly from strength-focused chair yoga since it enables them to gradually increase their muscle strength in a safe and regulated environment.

5. Chair Yoga for Restorative

The focus of restorative chair yoga is on stress relief and relaxation. To calm the nervous system and encourage relaxation, this type of yoga emphasizes deep breathing, meditation, and gentle stretches. Because it eases tension and encourages inner peace, restorative chair yoga is excellent for anyone dealing with stress, anxiety, or chronic pain.

It is common to practice restorative chair yoga poses slowly and for long periods. Seated Neck Stretches, Chair Pigeon Pose, and Seated Forward Fold are all useful for alleviating stiff muscles and encouraging relaxation. In restorative chair yoga sessions, breathing techniques including diaphragmatic breathing and alternate nostril breathing (Nadi Shodhana) are commonly utilized to help control the breath and release stress.

Because restorative chair yoga is gentle and emphasizes mental and emotional well-being in addition to physical activity, anyone can practice it, regardless of physical ability. It's a great way to help those who have trouble falling asleep, are anxious, or need a calming activity to decompress.

6. Yoga in Chairs for Balance

A key component of physical health is balance, particularly for older adults who are more prone to falls. Enhancing stability, coordination, and proprioception—the awareness of one's body's position in space—are the goals of chair yoga for balance. The postures in this chair yoga technique challenge the body's ability to stay upright while using the chair for support when necessary.

Seated Marching with Arm Swing, Chair Tree Pose, and Seated Chair Squat are designed to work the muscles involved in balance. Stability requires strength in the legs and core, which these exercises provide. People who regularly do chair yoga for balance may become more adept at moving with assurance and preventing falls.

In addition to being particularly beneficial for the elderly, balance-focused chair yoga can aid in the recovery of individuals whose coordination has been compromised by surgeries or accidents.

Everyone can benefit from chair yoga, whether their goal is to relax or improve their strength, flexibility, or balance. By choosing a chair yoga style that suits your particular objectives and physical capabilities, you may create a practice that enhances your health and well-being.

Overview Of Weight Loss And Its Advantages

Losing weight is often a complex issue that involves aspects of metabolism, food, exercise, and emotional health. Understanding the principles of weight reduction and its benefits is more important than ever in the modern world, when obesity rates are on the rise and health-related issues are becoming more prevalent. This study will shed light on the science behind weight loss and the numerous health advantages of keeping a healthy weight.

Fundamentally, weight loss happens when the body uses more energy than it takes in. The energy balance can be changed by several factors:

1. Creating a caloric deficit—that is, consuming fewer calories than your body needs to maintain its current weight—is the foundation of weight loss. The underlying math is simple: you will gain weight if you consume 2,500 calories a day but only burn 2,000 through physical activity and metabolic processes. You will lose weight if you consume 1,800 calories and burn 2,000.

2. The chemical process by which the body sustains life, including turning food into energy, is called metabolism. Because it indicates how many calories your body requires

at rest to carry out essential functions, basal metabolic rate, or BMR, is a crucial component of metabolism. Age, gender, muscle mass, and heredity are some of the elements that affect BMR, therefore depending on their metabolic rate, some people may find weight loss easier or more difficult.

3. By increasing calorie expenditure, exercise helps people lose weight. You can reduce weight by engaging in a variety of physical activities, from strength training to cardiovascular exercises like jogging, cycling, or walking. Additionally, because muscle burns more calories than fat, regular exercise can aid in the development of muscular mass, which raises metabolism.

4. Hormones play a significant role in both weight gain and loss. Leptin, ghrelin, cortisol, and insulin all have significant effects on metabolism, fat storage, and appetite control. Weight gain or trouble losing weight could result from an imbalance in these hormones. People can choose foods and lifestyles more wisely if they understand how these hormones function.

There are numerous physical and mental health advantages to losing extra weight. Among the most significant advantages are:

1. You can significantly lower your risk of developing chronic conditions including type 2 diabetes, heart disease, hypertension, and some types of cancer by maintaining a healthy weight. Being overweight puts stress on the body, which raises insulin resistance and inflammation—two things that increase the chance of developing chronic illnesses.

2. Losing weight can improve cholesterol, reduce blood pressure, and ease the strain on the heart. Maintaining a healthy weight can help reduce the risk of heart attacks and strokes by improving cardiac function and circulation.

3. Excessive weight can put undue strain on joints, especially weight-bearing joints like the hips and knees. This strain can be lessened by losing weight, which can increase mobility, reduce pain, and lower the risk of osteoarthritis.

4. Sleep apnea, a condition in which breathing stops momentarily while you sleep, is commonly linked to being overweight. These symptoms can be lessened with weight loss, improving sleep quality and general well-being.

5. Many people say they feel more alert and energized after losing weight. This energy boost can help with everyday chores, raise output, and promote an active lifestyle.

6. By boosting confidence and self-worth, weight loss can enhance mental health. Additionally, regular exercise, which is often linked to weight loss, releases endorphins, which can lessen anxiety and depressive symptoms.

7. A person's general quality of life can be enhanced by maintaining a healthier weight, which enables them to engage more fully in family, social, and recreational activities. It can offer a greater degree of contentment and well-being.

8. Studies have shown that maintaining a healthy weight is associated with a longer lifespan. Over time, losing weight can improve vitality and slow down the aging process.

Understanding the complex interactions between diet, exercise, metabolism, and psychology is essential to understanding weight loss. Beyond appearance, achieving and maintaining a healthy weight has many benefits, such as improved mental and physical health and a higher quality of life.

The Scientific Basis Of Chair Yoga And Loss Of Weight

For some who find traditional yoga practices too difficult or unavailable, chair yoga has emerged as a game-changing type of exercise. Examining the physiological, psychological, and behavioral aspects of chair yoga is necessary to comprehend the science behind the practice and how it affects weight loss.

Benefits of Chair Yoga for the Physiology

1. Metabolism and Caloric Burn: By boosting your calorie expenditure, chair yoga can aid in weight loss. Chair yoga considerably raises heart rate and metabolism, although it cannot burn as many calories as high-intensity exercises. When performed regularly, the mix of postures stretches, and motions can increase total energy expenditure. Studies have shown that even mild exercise can increase metabolic rates, which enables the body to burn fat for energy.

2. Strengthening and Activating Muscles: A range of positions that focus on different muscle groups make up chair yoga, which increases muscle strength and activation. For instance, exercises like the chair warrior and sitting leg raise improve both functional strength and muscle tone, both of which are necessary for day-to-day tasks. Because muscle burns more calories at rest than fat, gaining muscle is

particularly helpful for weight loss. Therefore, adding resistance through chair yoga encourages a metabolic environment that is conducive to weight loss.

3. increased Mobility and Flexibility: Maintaining an active lifestyle, particularly as we age, requires flexibility and agility. Chair yoga uses range-of-motion movements and mild stretching to improve flexibility. Better movement patterns and a decreased risk of injury can result from increased flexibility, which enables people to engage in additional physical activities that may help them lose weight. Additionally, greater mobility makes it possible for people to perform daily tasks more effectively, encouraging an active lifestyle that helps with weight management.

4. Stress Mitigation and Hormone Equilibrium: Because stress triggers the body's hormonal reactions, especially the production of cortisol, which is associated with the development of fat, it significantly affects weight regulation. Deep breathing and mindfulness are two relaxation methods that are included in chair yoga and can effectively lower stress levels. Regular relaxation techniques have been shown to reduce cortisol levels, which lessens the impact of stress on weight gain. Chair yoga's calming effects promote well-being, which supports weight loss initiatives.

Chair Yoga's Benefits for the Mind

1. Body Awareness & Mindfulness: By enabling practitioners to focus on their breathing, body sensations, and movements, chair yoga fosters awareness. A more deliberate approach to diet and lifestyle choices may arise from this heightened consciousness. Chair yoga strengthens the mind-body connection, which in turn encourages healthier eating habits. Research indicates that practicing mindfulness can result in better food choices and less emotional eating, both of which aid in weight loss.

2. Mental Health: By lessening the symptoms of worry and despair, which are commonly linked to weight gain, chair yoga can enhance mental health. Through movement, the practice fosters a positive environment where people can experience positive emotions and a sense of accomplishment. Higher self-esteem and motivation to reach weight loss objectives may arise from this emotional boost. Research indicates that individuals who integrate physical activity into their daily routine experience improved mood and a greater sense of self-efficacy, both of which contribute to weight loss.

Chair Yoga's Behavioral Aspects

1. Creating a Long-Term Habit: One of the most crucial elements of losing and maintaining weight loss is creating and maintaining a regular exercise routine. Because chair yoga is so accessible, people can incorporate it into their everyday routines with ease. People with physical restrictions can participate in daily activities without the obstacles that come with traditional workouts thanks to the option to practice while seated. People who develop the habit of practicing frequently might provide the foundation for successful weight loss in the long run.

2. Support & Community: The sense of support and community that chair yoga classes usually foster can encourage participants to stick with their weight loss objectives. Social connection and support are made possible by group membership, which strengthens positive behaviors. Research indicates that social support is a powerful indicator of weight loss program effectiveness. Chair yoga creates a positive atmosphere for personal growth by giving people a way to meet people who share their interests.

3. Empowerment via Flexibility: Chair yoga's adaptability to various fitness levels and physical conditions is one of its

unique selling points. Regardless of where they are coming from, this inclusivity empowers people to take control of their health and well-being. By providing adjustments and alternate positions, chair yoga encourages practitioners to pay attention to their bodies and progress at their own pace. This empowerment may lead to increased commitment to weight loss objectives and improved adherence to exercise regimens.

A powerful, scientifically supported weight-loss method that incorporates behavioral, psychological, and physiological elements is chair yoga. Chair yoga encourages calorie burning, muscle activation, flexibility, and stress reduction, all of which contribute to weight loss and overall health improvement. Chair yoga is a long-term option for anyone wishing to lose weight and improve their quality of life because of its mindfulness and community characteristics, which encourage healthy habits. Chair yoga will continue to play a significant role in the health and wellness scene as more people become aware of its advantages, proving that anyone can control their weight successfully, regardless of physical capabilities.

How Chair Yoga Enhances Flexibility And Movement

Maintaining flexibility and mobility is essential in today's more sedentary environment, particularly as we get older. Many people experience reduced range of motion and stiffness due to chronic health conditions, injuries, or inactivity. This is where chair yoga's advantages as a practice shine. People of all ages and abilities can perform yoga poses while seated using chair yoga.

It's critical to grasp the definitions of mobility and flexibility before delving into the specifics of chair yoga.

The capacity to move freely and effortlessly is known as mobility. Joint range of motion, coordination, and the capacity to carry out tasks comfortably are all included. Everyday activities like walking, bending, and getting out of a chair require good mobility.

Conversely, the capacity of muscles and tendons to stretch is known as flexibility. Being flexible allows joints to move freely, which is essential for physical activities. Increased flexibility can help with general physical health, athletic performance, and injury prevention.

The Value of Chair Yoga for Increasing Flexibility and Mobility

Chair yoga is a brand-new method of increasing flexibility and mobility that blends mindfulness and mindful breathing with mild exercises. It operates like this.

1. Gentle Movement: Chair yoga involves sitting in a chair or using it as support while performing a variety of poses. This makes it an excellent option for anyone who might find it challenging to perform standard yoga poses because of chronic pain, restricted mobility, or balance issues. Soft movements increase blood flow to muscles, alleviate stiff joints, and enhance overall body awareness.

2. Chair Yoga Pose: A lot of chair yoga poses are designed to be low-impact and good for your joints. People can engage their muscles and joints without placing them under stress, as standing positions do, by doing poses like the Chair Cat-Cow Stretch or Seated Mountain Pose. This gentle method encourages the necessary motions for improved flexibility and mobility while also reducing the risk of injury.

3. Focusing on Specific Muscle Groups: Chair yoga can be tailored to focus on specific muscle groups that are necessary for flexibility and mobility. For instance, postures that focus on the shoulders, hips, and lower back can

improve the range of motion and ease stress in these areas. The way these muscle groups function in daily duties can be greatly enhanced by regular chair yoga practice.

4. Enhanced Core Strength: A strong core is essential for maintaining stability and balance, two qualities that are essential for mobility. The core muscles are the focus of many chair yoga poses, which improve control and strength. Flexibility and core strength are strengthened with poses like the Seated Tummy Twist and Chair Warrior I, which improve overall mobility.

5. Better Balance: A key component of mobility is balance, and chair yoga offers a secure environment for honing balance-boosting skills. Situated postures such as Chair Tree Pose or Chair Warrior III, which assist develop the proprioceptive awareness necessary for stability and reducing the risk of falling, allow users to gradually challenge their balance while using the chair for support.

6. Chair yoga places a strong emphasis on the importance of breath awareness and control. The 4-4-4 breathing technique and deep belly breathing are useful for reducing stress and promoting relaxation. Our muscles are more likely to react favorably to stretching when we are relaxed, which increases our flexibility. Breath awareness also

enhances bodily awareness, enabling practitioners to pay attention to their bodies and adjust them as necessary.

7. Regular Practice and Consistency: One of the most important yoga precepts is consistency. Over time, chair yoga can help you become more flexible and mobile. People can try deeper stretches and increase their range of motion as they become more accustomed to the poses. People feel more empowered and are inspired to continue being active and involved in their daily lives as a result of this ongoing engagement with their bodies.

8. Mind-Body Connection: Chair yoga promotes a holistic approach to wellness by helping practitioners establish connections with their bodies and minds. People can identify areas of tightness and discomfort because of this mind-body connection, which heightens awareness of bodily sensations. Practitioners can modify poses to suit their needs and progress at their own pace by being aware of their bodies.

Chair Yoga Pose for Enhanced Flexibility and Mobility

Several chair yoga poses are excellent for increasing flexibility and mobility:

❖ Seated Mountain position: This fundamental pose promotes proper posture and core activation, which helps build stability and lengthens the spine.

❖ Chair Cat-Cow Stretch: This dynamic exercise relieves stress and warms the spine, resulting in increased neck and back flexibility.

❖ Seated Forward Bend: This pose helps to improve hip and spine flexibility by stretching the lower back and hamstrings.

❖ Chair Pigeon position: This position targets areas that are frequently stiff after extended sitting by opening the hips and extending the glutes.

❖ Chair Warrior poses: These poses enhance stability and balance, two essential elements of overall mobility while strengthening the legs.

People of all ages and capacities can benefit from chair yoga since it is a powerful practice that encourages flexibility and mobility. By combining gentle movements, mindful breathing, and an emphasis on body awareness, chair yoga enables practitioners to benefit from yoga's many health benefits while also enhancing their physical well-being. Chair yoga has the potential to revolutionize your wellness journey, regardless of your goals: reducing stiffness, increasing range of motion, or preserving your independence. With dedication and perseverance, chair yoga may improve your flexibility and mobility, leading to a more active and healthy lifestyle.

Low-Impact Movements' Benefits For People Of All Ages

Over the past few years, low-impact activities have gained popularity as an effective way to maintain physical health and well-being in individuals of all ages. These exercises are suitable for people of all ages, including beginners, the elderly, and those recovering from injuries, because they are well known for lowering joint tension and the risk of damage. The advantages of low-impact motions will be examined in this conversation, with a focus on their significance for all age groups.

1. Joint Well-being and Decreased Risk of Injury

The mildness of low-impact activities, which aids in joint protection, is one of its biggest advantages. Jogging, leaping, and other traditional high-impact exercises can cause serious strain on the ankles, hips, and knees. In older adults, this stress can worsen pre-existing joint issues, resulting in discomfort and limited movement. People can engage in physical activity without overtaxing their joints by doing low-impact exercises like chair yoga, cycling, and swimming. Because it encourages movement without exacerbating pain, this protective feature is particularly beneficial for people with arthritis or joint pain.

2. Better Cardiovascular Health

Cardiovascular health can be significantly enhanced by low-impact workouts. Low-impact aerobic exercises, walking, and cycling all work the heart and lungs without overtaxing them. Low-impact aerobic exercises can help lower blood pressure and cholesterol by increasing heart rate and enhancing circulation. For people of all ages, engaging in regular low-impact cardiovascular exercise is crucial to maintaining a healthy lifestyle because it reduces the risk of heart disease, stroke, and other cardiovascular illnesses.

3. Improved Balance and Flexibility

Low-impact activities may incorporate stretching and flexibility exercises to enhance range of motion and balance. For older people, who may become stiff and less flexible as they age, this is especially important. General mobility is enhanced by increased flexibility, which makes everyday activities like walking, bending, and reaching safer and easier. Additionally, while falls are a big problem for seniors, low-impact balancing exercises like yoga or tai chi may help reduce the risk. By encouraging better balance and coordination, these activities help people maintain their independence and self-confidence.

4. Controlling Weight and Increasing Metabolism

Additionally, low-impact exercise can support metabolism and weight control. Low-impact exercises can be sustained for extended periods, leading to a considerable calorie expenditure over time, whereas high-impact workouts burn more calories in less time. Low-impact exercises can also be easily incorporated into daily schedules, enabling people to be active without investing a lot of time. Taking the stairs rather than the elevator or walking rather than driving short distances can both improve metabolic function and weight management while also increasing overall physical activity.

5. Advantages for Mental Health

No matter how intense, physical activity has a big effect on mental health. Movements with little influence are not an exception. Frequent exercise releases endorphins, which are natural mood boosters that can help reduce melancholy and anxiety symptoms. In addition to fostering a sense of community and belonging, social interactions in group low-impact activities like chair yoga or dance can help older people feel less alone and lonely. Additionally, mindfulness practices like concentrating on movement and breath are commonly incorporated into low-impact workouts, which can enhance mental well-being and lower stress levels.

6. Inclusion and Accessibility

Accessibility is also another important benefit of low-impact workouts. Low-impact exercises are inclusive and can be customized to accommodate a range of fitness levels and physical conditions, in contrast to high-impact routines that may need certain skills or athletic aptitude. This flexibility makes it possible for those who are new to exercising, have chronic illnesses, or have impairments to participate safely and effectively. For instance, chair yoga makes it possible for elderly people and people with restricted mobility to strengthen and stretch while seated, guaranteeing that everyone has the chance to improve their physical well-being.

7. Promotion of Exercise Habits for Life

Exercise can be made more pleasurable rather than frightening by promoting a good attitude toward fitness through low-impact motions. People of all ages are encouraged to lead active lives by this strategy. When fitness regimens incorporate fun, low-impact activities like dancing, swimming, or gardening, people are more likely to maintain them. Long-term health advantages like longer lifespans, better quality of life, and a decreased chance of chronic illnesses can result from this dedication to regular exercise.

8. Improved Recuperation and Healing

Following surgery or an injury, low-impact exercises offer a safe means of regaining strength and mobility. To assist patients in recuperating without overtaxing their bodies, rehabilitation programs usually incorporate low-impact exercises. Exercises like swimming or cycling are often suggested by physical therapists as ways to strengthen muscles and enhance joint function. Exercise done gradually not only speeds up recovery but also lowers the chance of re-injury, enabling patients to confidently return to their regular activities.

9. Social Networks and Community Development

Group walking, chair yoga, and water aerobics are just a few of the low-impact movement activities that provide lots of chances for social interaction. These sessions can act as social gathering places for senior citizens, fostering camaraderie and a feeling of community. People are more likely to stick with their fitness adventures when they participate in low-impact workouts with others because it fosters motivation and accountability. Low-impact hobbies' social component can greatly enhance mental well-being and create a feeling of direction.

Lastly, Low-impact activities promote an inclusive environment for physical activity by emphasizing joint health, increasing cardiovascular fitness, improving flexibility and balance, bolstering mental well-being, and promoting accessibility. Incorporating low-impact activities into daily life, such as chair yoga, walking, or swimming, can improve quality of life, health outcomes, and the development of lifelong fitness habits. Understanding the importance of these mild yet effective exercises makes it clear that they are not just a fad but an essential part of everyone's healthy lifestyle, regardless of age or degree of fitness.

CHAPTER 2: BEGINNING YOUR CHAIR YOGA ADVENTURE

Selecting The Proper Chair And Accessories

Selecting the right chair and equipment is one of the most crucial elements of a fruitful chair yoga practice. Your chair yoga practice depends on the chair you select. When it comes to supporting your body throughout different exercises, not all chairs are made equal. Here are some essential characteristics to search for.

1. Robust design: Your chair needs to be sturdy and long-lasting. Seek to choose metal or wood chairs that are sturdy enough to hold more weight than you do. When doing workouts that require strength and balance, this ensures safely.

2. Seat Height: The chair's seat height is crucial. Your chair should support your knees at a 90-degree angle and your feet flat on the floor when you're seated. Try using a cushion to raise your sitting posture if you are unable to locate a chair that is the right height.

3. Seat Width and Depth: The seat should be sufficiently deep and wide to accommodate your body. You might not be able to perform different positions and feel uncomfortable if the seat is too shallow or narrow.

4. Back Support: For those with back issues, in particular, a chair with a supportive backrest is essential. To assist you in maintaining proper posture while practicing, look for chairs with lumbar support and a straight back.

5. Armrests: For some positions, chairs with armrests may offer additional support. To avoid limiting your range of motion during certain activities, make sure the armrests are not excessively high. Your arms should ideally slide under them with ease.

Chair Yoga Chairs:

Chair yoga often works well with regular office or dining chairs, but you can also look into specialty options:

1. Yoga Chairs: Designed especially for yoga, these chairs usually come with features that enhance your practice. They are appropriate for a range of exercises since they can have foldable designs, retractable backs, or changeable heights.

2. Stability Chairs: Designed to withstand dynamic motions, stability chairs offer extra support in more challenging positions. They usually incorporate extra components within their construction, including stability balls or resistance bands.

3. Foldable Chairs: Foldable chairs might be a fantastic choice for people who have little room for storage. Although they are portable and lightweight, they nevertheless need to adhere to the height and stability specifications.

Extra Tools to Help You Get Better at What You Do

The following add-ons could enhance your chair yoga practice in addition to the chair:

1. Yoga Mats: To improve stability and grip, place a yoga mat below your chair. This is particularly useful for chairs that might slip on tile or hardwood floors. Make sure the mat isn't slick to prevent accidents.

2. Cushions and bolsters: Cushions can be used to adjust height and offer extra comfort. For those who have trouble sitting upright, adding a cushion to the chair may help

maintain proper alignment. Additionally, the body can be supported in various positions with the use of braces.

3. Your chair yoga practice can become more varied and intense with the use of resistance bands. Because you can change the resistance level according to your abilities, they are particularly helpful for strength-building workouts.

4. Light Weights: You can enhance specific workouts and build strength without overtaxing your joints by using light dumbbells or wrist weights. Start with the smallest weight you can to prevent harm.

In many different postures, you can utilize yoga blocks to bring the ground closer to your body. They provide stability and support, which makes it easier to maintain proper alignment, particularly if your flexibility is limited.

Organizing Your Practice Area

Establishing a conducive atmosphere that encourages focus, relaxation, and physical well-being is essential when designing a chair yoga practice space. You may practice more efficiently and give each session your whole attention in a well-organized workspace. This is a comprehensive guide to setting up your space for chair yoga.

Selecting the Proper Site

Selecting the ideal location is the first step in setting up a chair yoga practice area. Find a quiet area in your house where you may practice without being bothered. This might be a distinct space, a nook in your living room, or even a bright spot on your porch.

Pick a place where there won't be any noise or distractions from family, pets, or electronics. Focus and relaxation require a peaceful environment. Choose a space that gets natural light if at all possible. You can feel happier and practice more effectively in the sun. Make sure it's easy to get to where you practice. It should be easy for you to get to, particularly if you have mobility problems.

Establishing a cozy setting

Your chair yoga experience will be significantly enhanced by creating a welcoming and cozy space. Make sure the temperature in the room is appropriate for your practice. You might want to adjust your air conditioning and heating systems or use blankets or fans as necessary. A calm mood can be produced with the use of soft, ambient lighting. Try using table or floor lamps with warm bulbs if there isn't enough natural light in your space. Steer clear of harsh overhead lights as it could be annoying.

Your mood can be significantly affected by scents. Think about using incense, candles, or essential oils to create a calming ambiance in your house. Citrus, eucalyptus, and lavender scents may aid in concentration and relaxation. Some people believe that practicing is aided by relaxing background music or ambient sounds. You have the option of guided meditation or quiet. Select something that makes you feel good and fosters a calm atmosphere.

Creating a schedule

Establishing a routine might help solidify your practice after your space is prepared. Select specific times of the week to practice chair yoga. You can develop a habit and fortify your commitment by being consistent. Take a moment to mentally prepare before every practice. To clear your head and focus your concentration, think about completing a quick meditation or deep breathing exercise.

Create a pre-practice routine to signal the start of your session. This can be taking a few deep breaths, lighting a candle, or playing a certain song. These routines help you redirect your attention from your everyday responsibilities to your yoga practice.

Adding Individual Touches

Your practice space might feel more inviting and significant if you add personal touches. Add things that inspire you, like pictures, plants, or artwork. These components may help create a lively and upbeat environment. You may enhance your practice space by bringing nature within. To promote relaxation and well-being, think of using flowers, plants, or other natural elements. To keep yourself motivated and goal-focused, put up motivational sayings or affirmations in your practice area.

The way you set up your chair yoga practice space is a personal choice that can greatly affect your results and experience. You may create a haven that supports your mind, body, and soul by carefully choosing the ideal spot, chair, and atmosphere, as well as by setting up your equipment. Recall that the ultimate objective of chair yoga is to cultivate a sense of calm, well-being, and self-connection in addition to physical conditioning. Enjoy the journey to improved fitness and health after taking the time to design an environment that meets your requirements and objectives.

Customizing Chair Yoga To Meet Personal Requirements And Capabilities

Chair yoga is a flexible activity that may be readily modified to accommodate each participant's needs and limitations. Chair yoga is a gentle yet efficient kind of exercise, regardless of whether you're dealing with age-related mobility problems, recovering from an injury, or managing a chronic illness. Because of its adaptability, it is perfect for seniors, those with disabilities, and anybody else searching for a low-impact exercise choice. We'll examine how to customize chair yoga to each person's abilities in this section, making it a secure and fulfilling practice.

Knowing your requirements and limitations is essential before embarking on a chair yoga trip. Your practice will be guided by this self-awareness, which will also allow you to make the necessary adjustments. Think about the following components:

1. Physical Limitations: Take into account any physical limitations you could have, such as joint issues, arthritis, decreased mobility, or chronic discomfort. The kinds of positions that are safe to do will depend on these factors.

2. Injury Recovery: If you are recovering from an injury, discuss safe and suitable movements with your physician or physical therapist.

3. Many people may have balance and coordination issues, especially the elderly. Being aware of these problems might assist you in selecting positions that lessen the risk of falling.

4. Flexibility: Everyone has varied levels of flexibility, which may affect how at ease you are in certain positions. Don't overdo it and pay attention to your body.

5. Energy Levels: Variations in your energy levels can be brought on by medication, illness, and fatigue. You can develop a regular practice routine by varying the length and intensity of your sessions.

Adapting the Chair Yoga Pose

Chair yoga is inherently adaptable, offering a variety of poses that may be customized to meet personal preferences. Chair yoga positions can be modified in the following ways:

1. Variations of Sat vs. Standing: Try a sat version if a posture, like the Warrior, is typically performed standing. Seated

Warrior I, for instance, can be executed by retaining the other hand on your hip while sitting upright in your chair and raising one arm overhead.

2. Use of Props: Your chair yoga practice can be significantly enhanced by the use of props. To support your body in different poses, use straps, pillows, or yoga blocks. For instance, to help deepen the stretch without straining, put a strap across the soles of your feet if you have problems reaching your feet during the Seated Forward Bend.

3. Changing the Range of Motion: Reduce the amount of movement your limbs can do if a position, like the Chair Pigeon posture, requires a wide range of motion. To feel a stretch, place your foot on the floor next to the opposing leg and slowly bend forward rather than crossing your ankle over your knee.

4. Pay Attention to Your Breath: In every chair yoga pose, breath is crucial. Focus on your breathing if you have trouble with a certain task. Deep, controlled breathing can help you relax and re-establish a connection with your body, even if you are unable to perform a full pose.

5. Slow Down: You may concentrate more on alignment and body awareness when you move more slowly. Take your

time if a series of positions seems overwhelming. Make sure you are secure and at ease in every position by holding each one for a few breaths before going on to the next.

Chair Yoga with Particular Restrictions

1. People with arthritis or other joint pain can benefit from chair yoga by becoming more flexible and less rigid. Focus on gentle motions that increase blood flow without causing pain. Choose seated stretches that focus on particular areas, such as the wrists and ankles, rather than poses that call for excessive bending or twisting.

2. Take into account sitting positions if your range of motion is restricted. Focus on simple stretches and strengthening exercises like chair glute bridges and seated leg lifts to build strength without standing. To guarantee a well-rounded practice, incorporate exercises that target the upper body and core.

3. Speak with your physician or physical therapist before beginning any exercise regimen after surgery. Start with easy chair yoga postures that build strength and flexibility without causing strain on the surgical area if you've been given the all-clear to exercise. Seated cat-cow and seated

hamstring stretches are two exercises that can help reduce tension and preserve mobility.

4. Energy swings can occur in people who have long-term conditions like fibromyalgia or chronic fatigue syndrome. Adapt your chair yoga routine to your energy level by incorporating more invigorating stretches when you're feeling up to it and more calming poses on days when you're feeling down. Allow for flexibility in your routine and pay attention to your body.

5. It's important to put stability first while practicing for people who have balance problems. Concentrate on sitting positions like Chair Warrior I and II that build core and leg strength. When doing seated actions that require additional stability or changing positions, think about leaning against a wall or other sturdy object for support.

The practice of awareness and listening to your body is one of the most crucial elements of customizing chair yoga to meet your needs. Be mindful of how each stance makes you feel, and don't be scared to modify or omit any awkward movements. Yoga is about finding what feels right for you, not about being perfectly aligned or looking a certain way.

Your experience is greatly influenced by the setting in which you practice. Establish a friendly and secure atmosphere. To provide a complete range of motion, make sure your chair is sturdy and armless. Use a nonstick surface or a yoga mat to prevent slippage. To help you focus on your breathing and movement, keep your surroundings clear of distractions.

To fully benefit from chair yoga, it is essential to modify the practice to match each person's needs and limitations. Chair yoga can be done safely and successfully provided you are aware of your unique challenges, modify your postures, and create a supportive environment. Strength, flexibility, and mindfulness can be developed at your rate because the goal of yoga is development rather than perfection. Chair yoga can be a useful tool for enhancing your overall health and quality of life with consistent practice.

Preparing For Chair Yoga Practices

A crucial component of any exercise regimen is warming up, and chair yoga is no different. Chair yoga is a safe and efficient way to increase flexibility, strength, and general well-being for a lot of people, especially seniors and those with limited mobility. Doing chair yoga without enough preparation, however, could lead to pain, strain, or injury, just like any other physical activity. For this reason, a carefully thought-out warm-up is essential.

Warming up serves several essential purposes:

1. Increases Blood Flow: A warm-up progressively increases blood circulation and heart rate, which enables oxygen and nutrients to get to your muscles. This process enhances overall performance and prepares your body for physical activity.

2. Enhances Flexibility: Warming up causes your muscles and joints to relax, which expands your range of motion and flexibility. Since many chair yoga poses call for the ability to gently stretch and bend, this is very crucial.

3. Lowers the Risk of Injury: By getting your body ready for exercise, a warm-up helps you avoid sprains and strains.

People with pre-existing illnesses and the elderly should pay particular attention to this.

4. Enhances Mental Focus: You can psychologically get ready for your practice by warming up. It enables you to transition from your daily activities to a more concentrated state, strengthening the mind-body connection—a crucial aspect of yoga.

5. Establishes the Tone for Practice: A warm-up can foster a calm environment that promotes mindfulness and relaxation. In chair yoga, where the emphasis is on self-awareness and gentle movements, this is very helpful.

Here are some excellent warm-up routines intended especially for chair yoga practitioners:

1. Gentle Sitting Movements:

❖ Neck Rolls: Start with sitting tall on your chair. Gently lower your chin to your chest while moving your head in a circular motion. Repeat for approximately 30 seconds in one direction before switching to the other.

❖ Shoulder Shrugs: Raise your shoulders to your ears, hold for a moment, and then lower. Repeat 5–10 times to alleviate shoulder tightness.

2. Arm and Wrist Stretches:

❖ Arm Circles: Extend your arms to the sides, making little circles. Gradually increase the size of the circles for approximately 30 seconds before switching directions.

❖ Wrist Rolls: Extend your arms in front of you with palms down. Rotate your wrists in circles for about 30 seconds before changing directions.

3. Spinal Warm-Up:

❖ Seated Cat-Cow Stretch: Sit up straight, hands on knees. As you breathe in, arch your back and look up (Cow Pose). As you exhale, curl your spine and tuck your chin (cat stance). Repeat this process for 5-10 breaths.

❖ Torso Twist: Sit upright with your right hand on the back of the chair. Inhale and stretch your spine, then exhale and twist slowly to the right, using your left hand for support. Hold for a few breaths, then switch sides.

4. Leg and Ankle Movement:

- ❖ Seated Leg Extensions: While sitting, straighten one leg while keeping the other foot flat on the ground. Hold for a few breaths, then switch legs. This warms up the quadriceps and promotes blood flow to the legs.

- ❖ Ankle Rotations: While sitting, lift one foot off the ground and rotate your ankle in circles for about 30 seconds. Switch directions and repeat with the other foot.

5. Breath Awareness:

Before going on to more active poses, take a moment to concentrate on your breathing. If you feel at ease, close your eyes and take a few deep belly breaths. Inhale via your nose, letting your abdomen rise, and exhale through your mouth. This strategy will help you relax and concentrate.

Warming up before chair yoga is an essential practice for improving both physical and mental readiness. A proper warm-up can help you achieve success in chair yoga by gradually increasing your heart rate, improving flexibility, and minimizing your risk of injury.

To maximize the benefits of your practice, incorporate gentle movements, stretches, and breath awareness into your warm-up regimen. Remember that chair yoga is all about finding ease and connection inside your own body, and a proper warm-up will help you get there. As you practice these warm-up movements, you'll be better equipped to reap the full benefits of chair yoga, paving the way for a healthier, more active lifestyle.

CHAPTER 3: BREATHING METHODS TO PROMOTE RELAXATION AND WEIGHT LOSS

Comprehending Pranayama

Life is a breath. It is essential to our health and fitness and is at the core of who we are. Even though we usually take it for granted, breathing is closely related to our mental, emotional, and physical well-being. The yoga method known as pranayama, which translates to ***"control of the life force"*** in Sanskrit, is used to carefully investigate this connection.

According to ancient texts like Patanjali's Yoga Sutras, pranayama is one of the eight limbs of yoga. It covers a range of breathing methods for managing and using the breath. In addition to inhaling and exhaling, pranayama emphasizes kumbhaka or the intervals between breaths. This all-encompassing approach emphasizes the breath as a means of boosting vitality and promoting mental and physical balance.

Pranayama's physiological effects are well known. By activating the parasympathetic nerve system, pranayama eases tension and encourages relaxation. Carefully adjusting breathing patterns can have an impact on blood pressure, heart rate, and overall metabolic function.

Certain pranayama techniques have been shown to enhance blood oxygenation, lung capacity, and respiratory system performance. Moreover, research indicates that pranayama may lower cortisol levels, the stress hormone, which promotes mental clarity and serenity.

The Advantages of Pranayama

1. Pranayama techniques promote calmness and aid in the reduction of tension and anxiety. People can better handle stress by breathing slowly and deliberately, which triggers the body's relaxation response.

2. By calming the mind and reducing distractions, pranayama enhances focus and concentration. Both professionals and students can benefit from this clarity since it can result in improved mental performance, attention, and concentration.

3. You may be able to better control your emotions by practicing breath control. By increasing self-awareness,

pranayama might help people better recognize and control their emotional reactions.

4. Consistent pranayama practice can lead to several health benefits, such as enhanced immune system performance, cardiovascular health, and digestion. It encourages the body to produce more oxygen, which is necessary for cellular function and general well-being.

5. By improving the passage of prana and oxygen, pranayama revitalizes the body. This surge of vitality can assist combat fatigue and improve general vitality.

6. A variety of pranayama techniques promote calmness and can aid in deeper, more restful sleep. An especially useful method for calming the mind before bed is Nadi Shodhana or alternating nostril breathing.

Methods of Pranayama

1. Diaphragmatic Breathing, also referred to as belly breathing, this method involves taking a deep breath through the nose and letting the diaphragm fully expand. This method expands lung capacity while promoting relaxation.

2. The "victorious breath," or ujjayi breath, is a technique that involves inhaling and exhaling via the nose while gradually constricting the throat to create a pleasing sound. This technique is commonly used to increase focus and produce heat internally during yoga practice.

3. Alternate nostril breathing, or Nadi Shodhana, is a practice that involves closing one nostril and taking a breath through the other before switching sides. By balancing the brain's left and right hemispheres, Nadi Shodhana promotes calmness and mental clarity.

4. The skull-shining breath, or kapalabhati, is characterized by quick, forceful exhalations that are followed by gentle inhalations. This energizing method helps to clear the mind and strengthens the respiratory system.

5. The Box Breathing (4-4-4) technique entails taking a four-count breath, holding it for four counts, letting it out for four counts, and then holding it out for another four counts. This method works particularly well for lowering anxiety and improving concentration.

6. The Bhramari (Bee Breath) method involves taking a deep breath and then humming as you exhale. Bhramari is

excellent for calming the mind and reducing tension and rage.

It can be easy and helpful to incorporate pranayama into your daily routine. *The following advice will help you get started:*

1. Every day, dedicate a short period of time to pranayama practice. This could be done in the evening to unwind or in the morning to start your day.

2. Seek out a quiet spot where you can sit comfortably and unhindered. Creating an atmosphere that encourages rest and focus is one way this helps.

3. When used with meditation, pranayama can improve the quality of your meditation. Practicing breath control first can help calm the mind and make it easier to enter a meditative state.

4. Consider how various strategies affect your emotions. Discover what works best for you because everyone reacts differently to pranayama.

5. In any discipline, consistency is crucial. More advantages and a stronger bond with your breath will come from consistent pranayama practice.

A powerful method that unites the mind, body, and soul is pranayama. We may enhance our mental clarity, emotional stability, and physical health by comprehending and controlling the power of breath. Your general health can be enhanced by including pranayama in your daily routine, regardless of your level of experience with yoga. Remember that the breath is ever-present, a continual reminder of the vigor and essence of life, as you study the various approaches and their advantages. Accept it and allow it to direct you toward harmony and well-being.

The Effects Of Breath On Stress Reduction, Metabolism, And Weight Loss

Although we usually take it for granted, breathing is an involuntary process that is essential to overall health, particularly in relation to metabolism, stress management, and weight loss. People's physical and emotional health can be enhanced by knowing how their breath works.

The exchange of carbon dioxide and oxygen between the organism and its environment occurs during breathing. Cellular metabolism, which turns food into energy, depends on oxygen. Oxygen enters the lungs during inhalation and binds to red blood cell hemoglobin. The various tissues and organs then receive this oxygen-rich blood to support metabolic functions. Conversely, when you exhale, the body releases carbon dioxide, which is a byproduct of metabolism.

The autonomic nervous system, which governs biological processes without conscious awareness, controls both the cardiovascular and respiratory systems. The parasympathetic neural system, which encourages rest and digestion activities, and the sympathetic nervous system, which regulates the "fight or flight" response, are the two branches of this system. By practicing mindful breathing techniques, people can affect these systems, as well as their metabolism and stress levels.

Inhalation and Energy Production

All biochemical processes that take place in the body, such as the breakdown of waste materials, the production of molecules, and the transformation of food into energy, are referred to as metabolism. Numerous metabolic pathways are impacted by breathing:

1. Oxygen Availability: For the best energy production, a healthy oxygen intake is necessary. Our metabolism functions better when our cells use oxygen more efficiently. Studies suggest that low oxygen levels may result in decreased metabolic rates, which would make losing weight more challenging.

2. Caloric expenditure can be increased by certain breathing techniques. For instance, deep, diaphragmatic breathing exercises help boost metabolism and lung capacity. These techniques are used in yoga and pilates, which enable practitioners to unwind and burn more calories.

3. Hormonal Regulation: Insulin and cortisol, two hormones that control metabolism, are released in response to

breathing. Insulin encourages cells to absorb glucose, but when cortisol, the stress hormone, is elevated over time, it can lead to fat storage. By managing their breathing and stress levels, people can better control these hormones, which supports a healthier metabolism.

Breathing and Losing Weight

Breathlessness and weight loss have a complex relationship. There are several ways in which practicing mindful breathing can aid with weight loss.

1. Eating Habits and Mindfulness: Yoga and meditation both involve mindful breathing techniques that can increase a person's awareness of their body and hunger signals. Deep, mindful breathing exercises before and during meals may help people become more conscious of their eating patterns, which in turn may reduce emotional and overeating tendencies.

2. Stress Reduction: Stress has a significant role in both weight gain and weight loss difficulties. The body produces cortisol in response to stress, which can increase cravings for unhealthy foods. The parasympathetic nervous system, which encourages relaxation and reduces cortisol levels, is

activated by deep breathing exercises. Weight loss and improved eating habits might result from reducing stress.

3. Improved Physical Performance: By improving endurance and physical performance, proper breathing techniques enable people to partake in more demanding activities. By raising calorie expenditure and promoting muscle growth, which improves metabolism, more physical activity can aid in weight loss.

Breathing Techniques to Reduce Stress

Breathing has a big effect on lowering tension. Prolonged stress can have negative effects on one's physical and emotional well-being, leading to depression, heart disease, and obesity.

Exercises involving deep breathing activate the parasympathetic nervous system by stimulating the vagus nerve. By reducing blood pressure and heart rate, this reaction mitigates the physiological effects of stress and encourages calm.

By focusing on the present, mindful breathing techniques help people detach from stressors and cultivate a sense of serenity. Stress-related anxiety and unpleasant thoughts can be reduced by concentrating on the breath.

Because breathing exercises let you process and let go of pent-up emotions, they can aid with emotional management. People who breathe deeply and intentionally are better able to control their responses to stimuli and develop more effective coping mechanisms.

One effective method for lowering stress, increasing metabolism, and losing weight is breathing. People can integrate useful breathing techniques into their daily routines and support a healthier lifestyle by being aware of the physiological and psychological consequences of breathing. Effective weight control and general well-being can result from learning the power of breath, whether through yoga, meditation, or conscious breathing techniques.

Diaphragmatic (Deep Belly) Breathing

Deep belly breathing, sometimes referred to as diaphragmatic breathing, is a breathing method that uses the diaphragm for intake and exhalation instead of the chest. In addition to encouraging relaxation, this breathing technique improves overall respiratory function and lung capacity. There are significant physical and mental health benefits to practicing diaphragmatic breathing in today's fast-paced environment, where shallow breathing has become the norm.

At the base of the thoracic cavity, the diaphragm is a dome-shaped muscle that divides the abdominal and chest cavities. It is necessary for respiration. The diaphragm contracts and slides downward during inhalation, enabling the lungs to fully expand. Consequently, the lower part of the lungs fills with air, which causes the muscles in the abdomen to contract and facilitates the exchange of oxygen. The diaphragm relaxes and forces air out of our lungs when we exhale.

The Importance of Deep Abdominal Breathing

1. By stimulating the parasympathetic nervous system, deep belly breathing lowers stress and encourages relaxation. Because it slows the heart rate and reduces cortisol, the stress hormone, this is particularly helpful for managing

stress and anxiety. Our bodies switch from the fight-or-flight response to a relaxed state when we take deep breaths.

2. Consistent diaphragmatic breathing increases lung capacity by strengthening the diaphragm. By concentrating on the upper chest, shallow breathing lowers the quantity of air that is efficiently inhaled and expended. Conversely, deep breathing fills the lungs more fully, improving oxygen exchange and guaranteeing that our bodies receive the oxygen they need to function.

3. By activating the diaphragm and abdominal muscles, deep belly breathing improves posture. We often adopt a slouched posture when we breathe shallowly, which over time can exacerbate musculoskeletal issues. By encouraging an upright posture, deep belly breathing helps to ease tension in the neck and back muscles and correct the spine.

4. Breathing diaphragmatically can aid in better digestion. By stimulating the abdominal organs, the diaphragm's movement enhances digestion and reduces discomfort and bloating. Since deep breathing can help calm the nervous system and encourage more efficient digestive processes, this is especially important for those who suffer from digestive issues brought on by stress.

5. By bringing our focus to our breath, deep belly breathing helps us become more conscious. This can be a useful tactic for keeping us rooted in the here and now. Focused breathing techniques can help clear the mind, get rid of distractions, and increase focus, which makes it simpler to tackle everyday tasks with clarity.

How to Breathe Deeply in the Belly

Whether you're lying down, doing chair yoga, or sitting at your computer, deep belly breathing is simple to include in your everyday routine. *Here is a detailed tutorial on how to become proficient in this method:*

1. To begin, settle into a cozy chair or lie down on your back. If you're sitting, maintain a straight back and flat feet on the ground. To support your lower back when you sleep on your side, place a cushion or pillow beneath your knees.

2. Two hands should be placed on your chest and abdomen, respectively. This will enable you to feel how your diaphragm moves while you breathe.

3. Slowly inhale via your nose, allowing the air to enter your abdomen instead of your chest. Imagine the balloon-like

expansion of your abdomen as it fills with air. For about four counts, try to take a deep, steady breath.

4. After you've taken a breath, hold it for about two counts. This time frame encourages relaxation and raises oxygen levels.

5. Breathe out gently through your lips, letting your stomach drop as you do so. Focus on letting your lungs empty. Aim for six counts for this exhale, which should be a little longer than the intake.

6. For a few minutes, keep doing this. Start with five to ten cycles, and as you become more comfortable with the method, progressively extend the duration.

7. Try to practice deep abdominal breathing many times a day. You can fit it into your daily schedule, work breaks, or bedtime wind-down routine.

Diaphragmatic breathing, another name for deep belly breathing, is a useful technique for enhancing overall health. By concentrating on the diaphragm, this technique enhances lung capacity, facilitates relaxation, improves posture, and supports digestive health. Deep belly breathing can help you regain emotional and physical control, lower stress levels, and increase awareness when included in your daily routine. You can benefit from this straightforward yet significant strategy with patience and effort, and pave the way for a better, more balanced life.

Box Breathing (4-4-4 Breathing Technique)

The 4-4-4 breathing method also referred to as box breathing, is a straightforward yet effective mindfulness exercise that promotes relaxation and lowers stress. This method creates a rhythmic pattern that resembles the four sides of a box by breathing, holding the breath, and exhaling for equal numbers. Athletes, members of the armed forces, and others seeking to enhance their mental and emotional well-being are among the professionals who employ box breathing.

Four equal parts, each lasting four counts, make up box breathing. This methodical approach aids in respiratory control, heart rate reduction, and the creation of a tranquil mood. The method is a flexible technique for managing stress and anxiety since it may be applied anywhere, at any time.

The Advantages of Box Breathing

1. The parasympathetic nervous system, which is triggered by box breathing, regulates the body's stress response. By slowing their breathing and concentrating on a regular pattern, people can lessen their stress and anxiety.

2. Box breathing's regularity helps to relax the mind, which facilitates task focus. When mental clarity is needed under duress, this might be extremely helpful.

3. People who practice box breathing are better able to manage their emotions. By allowing a pause between breaths, people can react to situations more thoughtfully rather than rashly.

4. By practicing box breathing before bed, you can help your body tell you when it's time to unwind. This technique can improve sleep quality and relaxation, which makes it easier to reach a calm condition.

5. By concentrating on the breath, box breathing encourages presence and awareness. By focusing on the here and now, people can become more conscious of their thoughts and emotions and feel more connected to both their surroundings and themselves.

How to Use the Breathing Method known as 4-4-4

The 4-4-4 breathing technique is easy to practice and may be done anywhere, including at home, at work, or even during a hectic day's break. To help you get started, here is a detailed tutorial:

1. Take a comfortable seat with your back straight in a chair or on the floor. If lying down is more comfortable, you can do it as well. Make sure your hands are on your lap or thighs.

2. Shutting your eyes can help you concentrate on your breathing and block out distractions. Keep your eyes slightly open and concentrate on a stationary object in front of you, if you'd like.

3. Take a deep inhale through your nose for four counts to begin. As you inhale, concentrate on filling your lungs and letting your belly grow.

4. Hold your breath for four more counts after you've finished breathing. Give your body time to unwind and focus on whatever feelings it may be having

5. Take a leisurely, four-count breath through your mouth. Release any tension or stress by taking a deep breath out.

6. Hold your breath for four more counts once you've released it. Make the most of this time by being mindful of your feelings and in the moment.

7. For a few minutes, keep using this method. Try to complete at least five cycles, gradually extending the time as you become more comfortable with the method.

The 4-4-4 breathing method sometimes referred to as box breathing, is a successful stress-reduction strategy that enhances concentration and fosters mental health. Its methodical approach to breath control helps people become more calm and more present, which makes it a useful exercise for anyone trying to become more emotionally resilient and mentally clear. You can live a better, more balanced existence and experience major benefits by incorporating box breathing into your daily routine. Regardless of your level of experience, box breathing is an easy and efficient method to enhance your overall health.

Inhaling Through Different Nostrils (Nadi Shodhana)

A classic yogic method called alternate nostril breathing, or Nadi Shodhana in Sanskrit, balances the body's energy pathways and encourages relaxation and mental clarity. To balance the left and right hemispheres of the brain, this breathing technique alternates the passage of breath between the left and right nostrils. With origins in ancient Indian philosophy, Nadi Shodhana is a well-liked yoga and meditation method for enhancing both mental and physical well-being.

According to the theory behind Nadi Shodhana, our bodies have energy channels called "nadis." The Ida, Pingala, and Sushumna are three of the body's hundreds of nadis that are particularly significant. The moon's soothing, cooling energy (yin) is associated with the Ida nadi, which flows down the left side of the body, while the sun's dynamic, heating energy (yang) is associated with the Pingala nadi, which runs down the right side. The path of spiritual energy (kundalini) is represented by the Sushumna nadi, which is positioned in the center.

By balancing the Ida and Pingala nadis' energies, alternate nostril breathing helps to maintain mental and physical equilibrium. This method lowers stress, enhances concentration, and fosters emotional stability.

Benefits of Inhaling through Alternate Nostrils

1. By calming the nervous system, Nadi Shodhana lessens tension and anxiety. By concentrating on the breath and creating a rhythmic pattern, this exercise encourages calm and relaxation.

2. Alternating nostril breathing enhances mental clarity and cognitive function by balancing the left and right hemispheres of the brain. For those who struggle to focus or have brain fog, it works wonders.

3. By balancing the body's energies, the exercise encourages emotional stability. People may respond to stimuli more composedly and have better emotional control as a result.

4. Deep, conscious breathing is encouraged by Nadi Shodhana, which may enhance respiratory function and lung capacity. This technique promotes a more effective carbon dioxide and oxygen exchange, which enhances overall health.

5. One useful technique for preparing the mind for meditation is alternate nostril breathing. It makes it easier to enter a meditative state by enhancing presence and focus.

Methods for Alternating Nostril Breathing Practice

The straightforward practice of Nadi Shodhana can be performed anywhere, including on the floor, in a chair, or even while lying down. To help you get started, here is a detailed tutorial:

1. Place your feet flat on the floor and sit comfortably cross-legged on the floor or in a chair. Maintain a straight back and relaxed shoulders.

2. Take a few deep breaths and gently close your eyes to help you center yourself. Breathe easily as you bring your attention to the here and now.

3. For this exercise, use your right hand. You have two options: alternate nostrils with your thumb and ring finger or extend your index and middle fingers and position them between your brows.

   1. To close the right nostril, use the thumb.
   2. The left nostril is sealed with the ring finger.

4. Start by taking a deep breath through your left nostril and using your thumb to seal your right nostril. Focus on getting your lungs full.

5. After taking a breath, close your left nostril with your ring finger and open your right. If it feels comfortable, hold your breath for a little moment.

6. Slowly and fully exhale via your right nostril. Try to release any tension or stress as you exhale.

7. Next, close your left nostril with your ring finger and take a big breath through your right.

8. After taking a breath, close your right nostril with your thumb and open your left. Hold your breath for a moment if you are comfortable doing so.

9. Take a deep, leisurely breath out of your left nostril. One cycle has therefore finished.

10. For five to ten minutes, repeat this cycle while maintaining steady, peaceful breathing. Breathe evenly and smoothly so that your body can adjust to the rhythm.

Nadi Shodhana, or alternate nostril breathing, is a very powerful technique for fostering mental clarity, balance, and relaxation. This method balances the body's energy pathways, which lowers stress, increases focus, and promotes emotional stability. There are many advantages to Nadi Shodhana, whether you're looking to improve your meditation skills or just find a calming pastime to incorporate into your daily schedule. The door to a happier, more balanced existence may be opened by using the power of your breath to foster greater well-being and connection with yourself with consistent practice.

The physical and mental benefits of chair yoga are increased when breathing techniques are used, leading to a more comprehensive approach to wellbeing. Practitioners can strengthen their bond with their bodies, lower stress levels, and encourage relaxation by concentrating on their breathing. Tell them that breathing is a path to inner peace and mindfulness as well as a means of movement while they do chair yoga. Chair yoga can become a life-changing activity that enhances their general quality of life if this awareness is developed.

CHAPTER 4: CHAIR YOGA WORKOUTS TO LOSE WEIGHT

---

1. Tadasana (seated mountain pose)

Instructions:

1. Sit upright, feet flat on the floor, and spine straight.
2. Place your hands on your thighs or lap.
3. Inhale deeply, elevating your chest and extending your spine.
4. Raise your arms, palms facing each other or clasped above your head.
5. Hold for 30-60 seconds, taking deep breaths and then exhaling to relax your arms.

Benefits:

❖ Improves posture and spinal alignment.
❖ Relaxes the mind and increases attention.

2. Chair Cat-Cow Stretch

Instructions:

1. Sit in a chair, feet flat on the ground, hands on knees.
2. As you breathe in, arch your back and raise your chest to the ceiling (Cow Pose).
3. As you exhale, curl your spine and tuck your chin into your chest (Cat Pose).
4. Repeat the movements for a few breaths.

Benefits:

* Enhances spinal flexibility and mobility.
* Reduces stress in the back and neck.

3. Seated forward bend (Paschimottanasana).

Instructions:

1. Sit with your feet flat on the ground and your knees slightly bent.
2. Inhale to lengthen your spine; exhale to bend forward from your hips.
3. Stretch your back and hamstrings by lowering your hands or feet to the floor.

4. Hold for a few breaths before returning to an upright
   position.

Benefits:

❖ Stretches the hamstrings and lower back.
❖ Helps to reduce tension and relax the mind.

4. Chair in extended side angle pose

Instructions:

1. Sit upright, with your feet planted.
2. Inhale and raise your right arm overhead.
3. Exhale and bend to the left, placing your left hand on the
   seat or thigh to generate a side stretch.
4. Hold for a few breaths, then switch sides.

Benefits:

❖ Stretches the side body and improves balance.
❖ Increases flexibility in the spine and hips.

5. Seated Spinal Twist (Ardha Matsyendrasana)

Instructions:

1. Sit tall, feet flat on the ground.
2. Inhale and straighten your spine.
3. On the exhale, twist your torso to the right, bringing your left hand to your right knee and your right hand behind you on the chair.
4. Hold for a few breaths, then switch sides.

Benefits:

❖ Improves spinal mobility and digestion.
❖ Reduces lower-back tightness.

6. Chair Pigeon Pose (Figure 4-Stretch)

Instructions:

1. Sit with your feet flat on the floor.
2. Cross your right ankle over your left knee, forming a figure-four shape.
3. To stretch your hips, softly press your right knee down toward the ground.
4. Hold for a few breaths, then switch sides.

Benefits:

- ❖ Hip and gluteal opening and extension.
- ❖ Reduces lower back and hip stress.

7. Seated leg raises

Instructions:

1. Sit with your back straight and your feet flat on the floor.
2. Lift one leg straight ahead of you and hold for a few seconds before lowering it back down.
3. Repeat multiple rounds with alternating legs.

Benefits:

- ❖ It strengthens the quadriceps and core.
- ❖ Improves lower-body mobility.

8. Chair Warrior I

Instructions:

1. Sit on the chair's edge, right foot forward and left foot back in a lunge position.

2. Raise your arms, palms facing each other.
3. Hold for a few breaths, then switch sides.

Benefits:

❖ Strengthens the legs and stretches the hips.
❖ Improves balance and stability.

9. Chair Warrior 2

Instructions:

1. Extend your arms parallel to the floor, one forward and one back, palms facing down.
2. Turn your head to check your front hand.
3. Hold for a few breaths, then switch sides.

Benefits:

❖ It strengthens both the legs and the core.
❖ Enhances focus and concentration.

10. Chair Warrior III

Instructions:

1. Sit with your feet planted.
2. Lean slightly forward, elevate your left leg behind you, and stretch your arms forward for balance.
3. Hold for a few breaths, then switch legs.

Benefits:

* ❖ Strengthens the core and legs.
* ❖ Improves balance and coordination.

11. Seated Chair Squat

Instructions:

1. Sit on the edge of a sturdy chair, your feet hip-width apart and securely planted on the floor.
2. Engage your core, and while keeping your chest upright, push through your heels to lift your body to a standing position.
3. Slowly lower yourself back down, very lightly touching the chair with your hips before standing back up. Repeat a few times.

Benefits:

❖ The quadriceps, glutes, and hamstrings are strengthened, which improves lower-body strength and mobility.
❖ Improves balance and stability, reducing the risk of falling.

12. Seated Tummy Twist

Instructions:

1. Sit in the chair with your feet flat on the ground.
2. Tighten your core and place your hands on your knees.
3. Twist your torso to the right, putting your left palm on your right knee and holding for a few breaths.
4. Repeat for the other side.

Benefits:

❖ Improves spinal flexibility and mobility.
❖ Strengthens the oblique muscles, improving core stability.

13. Chair Sun Salutation

Instructions:

1. Begin by sitting upright in a chair, feet flat on the floor.
2. Inhale and raise your arms aloft in an upward salute.
3. Exhale and fold forward, bringing your hands to your feet.
4. Inhale, return to a seated position and lift your arms again.

Benefits:

❖ Increases flexibility, especially in the spine and hamstrings.
❖ Enhances circulation and warms the body.

14. Seated Marching

Instructions:

1. Sit upright in a chair, feet flat on the floor.
2. Lift your right knee to your chest, then lower it.
3. Continue on the left side, alternating legs as if marching.

Benefits:

❖ Gentle movement improves cardiovascular health.
❖ Strengthens hip flexors and improves coordination.

15. Chair Hip Stretch

1. Sit in the chair with your right ankle crossed over your left knee, producing a figure-four shape.
2. Lean slightly forward to lengthen the stretch in your right hip.
3. Pause for a few breaths before swapping sides.

Benefits:

❖ Reduces tension on the hips and lower back.
❖ Improves hip muscle flexibility.

16. Seated Knee Lifts

Instructions:

1. Sit tall in a chair, feet flat on the floor.
2. Engage your core by bringing one knee to your chest.
3. Lower one leg and repeat on the other side, alternating legs.

Benefits:

❖ It strengthens the lower abdominal muscles.

❖ Enhances hip mobility and lower-body coordination.

17. Chair Leg Extensions

Instructions:

1. Sit in the chair, back straight, feet level with the ground.
2. Lift your right leg straight out in front of you and hold for a few seconds before lowering it back down.
3. Repeat with the left leg.

Benefits:

❖ Strengthens the quadriceps and improves knee joint health.
❖ Improves lower-body endurance and stability.

18. Seated Hamstring Stretch

Instructions:

1. Sit on the edge of a chair, with one leg extended in front of you and your heel on the ground.
2. Lean forward from the hips, keeping your back straight and focusing on your toes.
3. Hold the stretch, then switch sides.

Benefits:

- ❖ Stretches the hamstrings and lower back.
- ❖ Reduces tension and promotes good posture.

19. Seated Crescent Moon Pose

Instructions:

1. Sit upright with your feet level with the ground.
2. Inhale and raise both arms aloft.
3. Exhale and bend to the right, extending your left arm above your head.
4. Hold and repeat on the other side.

Benefits:

- ❖ Stretches the sides of the body and improves spinal flexibility.
- ❖ Improves core stability and balance.

20. Chair Star Pose

Instructions:

1. Sit in the chair with your feet apart.
2. Extend both arms to the sides, creating a star shape with your body.
3. Pause for a few breaths before lowering your arms.

Benefits:

❖ Improves general posture and shoulder mobility.
❖ It strengthens the back muscles and widens the chest.

21. Seated Bicycle Crunches

Instructions:

1. Sit on the edge of a chair, back straight.
2. Lift your right knee to your chest, then twist your torso to bring your left elbow to your knee.
3. Switch sides and do several reps.

Benefits:

- ❖ Strengthens abdominal muscles and enhances core stability.
- ❖ Enhances coordination and balance.

22. Chair Floating Stick Pose

Instructions:

1. Sit on the edge of the chair, with your feet flat on the floor.
2. Using your core, lift both legs straight out in front of you.
3. Stretch your arms forward, parallel to the ground, and hold for a few breaths.

Benefits:

- ❖ Strengthens core muscles and improves posture.
- ❖ Enhances balance and stability.

23. Seated eagle pose

Instructions:

1. Sit erect in a chair, feet level with the ground.
2. Cross your right thigh over your left, then bring your right arm under your left, wrapping around your elbows.
3. Maintain your position and repeat on the opposing side.

Benefits:

❖ Stretches the shoulders and hips for increased flexibility.
❖ Improves concentration and balance.

24. Chair Neck Stretch

Instructions:

1. Sit comfortably with your feet flat on the ground.
2. Gently tilt your head to the right, bringing your ear to your shoulder.
3. Pause for a few breaths before swapping sides.

Benefits:

- ❖ Reduces stress in the neck and upper back.
- ❖ Increases cervical spine mobility.

25. Seated Wrist and Finger Stretches

Instructions:

1. Sit with your feet flat and one arm stretched out in front of you.
2. With your other hand, gently pull your fingers back to stretch the wrist.
3. Repeat with both hands.

Benefits:

- ❖ Improves wrist and finger flexibility.
- ❖ Reduces the tension and stiffness induced by repeated activities.

26. Seated Ankle Rotations

Instructions:

1. Sit tall with your feet flat on the ground.
2. Lift one foot off the ground and spin the ankle in clockwise and counterclockwise directions.
3. Repeat for the other foot.

Benefits:

❖ Improves ankle flexibility and mobility.
❖ Improves the circulation in the lower legs.

27. Chair Low Boat Pose

Instructions:

1. Sit with your hands on the chair's edges.
2. Lean back slightly and raise your legs straight.
3. Hold for a few breaths.

Benefits:

❖ Strengthens the core, specifically the lower abdominal muscles.

❖ Improves overall balance and stability.

28. Seated Camel Pose

Instructions:

1. Sit on the edge of a chair, feet level on the ground.
2. Place your hands on the back of the chair, arching your back and expanding your chest.
3. Pause for a few breaths before releasing.

Benefits:

❖ Expands the chest and expands the front of the body.
❖ Increases spinal flexibility while reducing lower back tightness.

29. Chair Core Twist

Instructions:

1. Sit upright with your feet level with the ground.
2. Cross your arms over your chest, then twist to one side, allowing your core to move.
3. Take a few breaths, then repeat on the opposite side.

Benefits:

- ❖ Strengthens the oblique muscles, which improves core stability.
- ❖ Increases spinal flexibility.

30. Seated Oblique Bend

Instructions:

1. Sit up straight, feet flat on the ground, arms aloft.
2. Lean to one side and raise the other arm up, feeling the stretch along your side.
3. Hold and switch the sides.

Benefits:

- ❖ The obliques are strengthened and extended.
- ❖ Improves balance and spinal flexibility.

31. Chair Tree Pose

Instructions:

1. Sit tall on your chair, feet flat on the floor.
2. Place your right foot against the inside thigh of your left leg.
3. Hold your hands in a prayer position before switching sides.

Benefits:

❖ Improves balance and coordination.
❖ It strengthens both the legs and the core.

32. Seated March with Arm Swing.

Instructions:

1. Sit upright with your feet level with the ground.
2. Lift one knee at a time, as if marching, and swing your arms in the opposite direction as your legs.
3. Perform several repetitions.

Benefits:

❖ Enhances cardiovascular function and coordination.
❖ Strengthens the hip flexors and increases joint mobility.

33. Chair Glute Bridge

Instructions:

1. Sit at the edge of the chair, hands on the seat.
2. Slide your feet forward and raise your hips, holding your glutes, before lowering.
3. Repeat several times.

Benefits:

❖ Strengthens the glute and hamstring muscles.
❖ Enhances lower-body stability and mobility.

34. Seated Chair Tappers

Instructions:

1. Sit upright with your feet slightly apart.
2. Reach your arms forward and alternately tap your feet on the floor, quickly raising them.
3. Continue for a few repetitions.

Benefits:

❖ Increases cardiovascular endurance.
❖ Improves foot and leg coordination.

35. Chair Reverse Plank

Instructions:

1. Sit on the edge of the chair, grasping the edges.
2. Use your arms to raise your hips and extend your legs forward.
3. Hold for a few breaths.

Benefits:

❖ It strengthens the arms, core, and glutes.
❖ Improves overall stability and coordination.

36. Seated Toe Taps

Instructions:

1. Sit upright and lift one foot off the ground slightly.
2. Tap your toes on the floor, rapidly rising and descending.
3. Repeat on the other side.

Benefits:

- ❖ Strengthens the calves and improves foot flexibility.
- ❖ Enhances coordination and circulation.

37. Seated Arm Circles

Instructions:

1. Sit up straight with your arms extended to the sides.
2. Move your arms in little circular motions, then reverse direction.
3. Continue for a few repetitions.

Benefits:

- ❖ Strengthens and stabilizes the shoulder joints.
- ❖ It enhances upper-body mobility and flexibility.

38. Push-ups with a chair seat

Instructions:

1. Stand behind the chair and place your hands on the seat.
2. Take a short step back and do a push-up with your elbows bent and your chest down to the seat.
3. Push back up to the starting position and repeat.

Benefits:

❖ It strengthens the chest, shoulders, and triceps.
❖ Improves upper-body endurance and stability.

39. Seated scissor kicks

Instructions:

1. Sit upright and grasp the chair's sides.
2. Extend both legs out in front of you and alternatively cross them over each other, as if making scissor motions.
3. Continue for a few repetitions.

Benefits:

- ❖ It strengthens the lower abdominal muscles.
- ❖ Improves hip and leg flexibility.

CHAPTER 5: ADAPTING CHAIR YOGA TO VARIOUS LEVELS OF FITNESS

Chair Yoga Adaptations For Beginners, Intermediate, And Experienced Practitioners

Knowing how to adjust postures and routines according to your skill level is essential as you embark on your chair yoga journey. By enabling you to gradually increase your strength, flexibility, and confidence, this technique not only guarantees safety but also enhances your practice.

Understanding Your Starting Point

❖ **Beginners:** The aim should be to establish a solid foundation if chair yoga or exercise in general is new to you. Start with easy poses and movements to increase your body awareness and teach you the basics of yoga. It's important to pay attention to your body and refrain from overexerting oneself, as this could cause harm or discomfort.

❖ ***Intermediates:*** People with a basic understanding of chair yoga or fitness, in general, can experiment with new poses and add increasingly challenging exercises. This level permits experimenting with different approaches to enhance flexibility, strength, and balance while preserving alignment and safety.

❖ ***Advanced Practitioners:*** You can go on to increasingly difficult poses and transitions after you've mastered chair yoga and built a strong foundation. In order to enhance your overall experience, this level encourages a more thorough analysis of breath work, sophisticated alignment methods, and the introduction of mindfulness exercises.

Chair Yoga Adapted for Beginners

1. Focus on basic poses that enhance flexibility and strength without taxing the body excessively.
2. To make positions more approachable, beginners should make adjustments.
3. Develop the ability to link breathing and movement. Deep belly breathing is one of the easy breathing exercises that can help you feel calmer and more centered. Your practice is more productive overall because of this relationship.
4. As a beginner, make practice sessions short and doable. Try to do chair yoga for 15 to 20 minutes, holding each pose for

three to five breaths. Increase the duration gradually as you become more at ease.

5. Help beginners respect their bodies and promote self-awareness. Change your posture or stay away from anything that hurts.

Modifying Chair Yoga for Intermediate

1. Intermediate practitioners can begin adding more diverse poses to their routines.
2. Include variations that will put your strength and balance to the test. For instance, you can increase the stretch and engagement of your core by extending your arms out to the sides during the Chair Warrior II.
3. Flow sequences that incorporate a variety of positions may be beneficial for intermediate practitioners.
4. As you progress, focus more on breathing control and alignment. You can create a rhythm and maintain focus during your practice by using breathing exercises like 4-4-4 Breathing (Box Breathing).
5. Increase your practice time gradually to 30 to 45 minutes so that you can incorporate additional poses and transitions. Strength and endurance will both be improved by this increase.

Chair Yoga Adaptation for Experienced Practitioners

1. Skilled practitioners are able to try out challenging poses that call for concentration, strength, and balance.
2. Try poses like Chair Tree Pose that need more balance. Instead of placing the foot on the thigh, place it on the ankle or calf to change the position.
3. Body scans and meditation are two methods that advanced practitioners can use to incorporate awareness into their practice. These methods improve the connection between the mind and body and raise self-awareness.
4. Try other chair yoga styles or add elements from other disciplines, such as Tai Chi or Pilates, to mix up your routine and challenge your body in novel ways.
5. Challenge yourself by establishing objectives like extending a posture, improving your flexibility, or trying out novel sequences. To record your progress and reflect on your experiences, keep a journal.

For a safe and effective practice, chair yoga must be modified for beginners, intermediates, and experts. Each practitioner can benefit from chair yoga's many benefits, including improved strength, flexibility, and general well-being, by customizing poses to suit their needs and gradually increasing the level of difficulty. Chair yoga provides a special chance to enhance your mental and physical well-being while accommodating different fitness levels, regardless of your degree of experience. Be patient with yourself, pay attention to your body, and relish the journey to improved fitness and health.

How Chair Yoga Can Help You Advance Safely

1. Recognize Your Present Capability

Examine your current mobility and health before starting your chair yoga practice. Think about this.

- ❖ Physical limitations: Look for any physical limitations, such as balance issues, joint pain, or muscular weakness. You can select the ideal positions and adjustments by being aware of these factors.
- ❖ Previous Experience: Consider your past experiences with yoga or fitness. Before moving on to more intricate versions, beginners should begin with basic chair yoga poses.
- ❖ Medical Conditions: See a healthcare professional if you have any health issues that might make it difficult for you to do chair yoga. They can provide guidance tailored to your particular needs.

2. Lay a strong foundation first

Make sure you have a solid basis before attempting to grow your practice. This comprises:

❖ Learn the fundamental poses: including the Seated Forward Bend, Chair Cat-Cow Stretch, and Seated Mountain Pose. Gaining confidence and stability can be achieved by becoming proficient in these positions.

❖ Increasing Flexibility and Strength: To improve your general strength and flexibility, use gentle movements and stretches. Regularly performing simple chair yoga poses will create a solid foundation for future development.

3. Pay attention to your body

To advance in chair yoga safely, you must pay attention to your body. Be mindful of the following:

❖ Body Signals: During and after practice, pay attention to how your body feels. If you are tired, in pain, or uncomfortable, change your strategy or take a break as necessary.

❖ Limitations: Be mindful of your limitations and refrain from stepping outside of your comfort zone. Pay attention to what your body is telling you and adjust as necessary.

4. Increase the difficulty gradually

Increase the difficulty of your practice gradually as you become more comfortable with basic poses:

❖ Introduce New Positions: Start introducing new, marginally more challenging positions after you have a firm grasp of the basic ones. Chair Warrior I and Chair Pigeon Pose are two examples.

❖ Adjust Current postures: Try out different iterations of postures you are familiar with as your confidence increases. For instance, to increase your strength and balance when performing Chair Warrior II, extend your arms out to the side.

❖ Boost Repetitions and Duration: Increase the length of your practice overall and the time of each pose gradually. As your endurance increases, increase the duration of your workouts from 15 to 20 minutes to 30 to 45 minutes.

5. Include Breathing exercises

An essential component of yoga, breathwork can help you advance your practice.

❖ Breath Awareness: Maintain a steady, deep breath throughout each pose. This link between movement and breath encourages serenity and improves the quality of practice as a whole.

❖ Present Breathing Methods: Include breathing exercises such as diaphragmatic breathing or 4-4-4 breathing (box breathing) in your regimen. These methods can increase your level of relaxation and enjoyment of your yoga practice.

6. Establish reasonable objectives

Establishing realistic objectives could direct your chair yoga development.

❖ Short-Term Objectives: Establish short-term objectives for particular abilities or advancements, such as learning a new posture or maintaining a stance for an extended period.
❖ Long-Term Objectives: Establish long-term objectives for your overall health and welfare. This can entail strengthening your muscles, improving your flexibility, or including chair yoga in your routine.

7. Use relaxation and mindfulness practices

As you progress, think about fusing relaxation and mindfulness practices to enhance your overall experience.

❖ Mindfulness Techniques: Concentrate on the here and now and develop an awareness of your body and breath to integrate mindfulness into your chair yoga practice.

❖ Guided Meditations: To enhance mental clarity and emotional well-being, conclude your practice with guided meditations or relaxation exercises.

8. Seek advice and assistance from the community

Participating in a community or asking for help could help you get better at chair yoga.

❖ Think about going to a certified instructor-led chair yoga class. As you develop, they can provide tailored guidance, adjustments, and assistance.
❖ To expand your practice and pick up new poses and sequences, use online resources such as movies or online courses.

9. Acknowledge development and adjust

Acknowledging and applauding your accomplishments is essential for motivation.

❖ Recognize Success: Honor each accomplishment, no matter how small. Acknowledging your progress will help you stay motivated, whether it's learning a new pose or extending your practice time.

❖ Modify as necessary: Because life conditions can vary, it's important to adjust your practice accordingly. Adjust your strategy and go back to the fundamental positions as necessary if you run into additional limitations or issues.

To properly advance with chair yoga, you must first learn about your body, then establish a solid foundation and gradually increase the level of difficulty while paying attention to your body's signals. You may enhance your chair yoga practice and benefit from its numerous benefits by including mindfulness, establishing realistic goals, and getting guidance. Keep in mind that learning yoga is a personal journey that calls for perseverance, self-compassion, and patience. Savor and value every stage of your chair yoga practice.

CHAPTER 6: MEAL PLANNING AND NUTRITION FOR WEIGHT LOSS

Being Aware Of How Nutrition Affects Weight Loss

Losing weight is a complex process that calls for many lifestyle changes, with diet being a key component. Exercise is essential for burning calories and improving overall fitness, but our ability to lose weight effectively and sustainably is directly impacted by the foods we eat.

People must attain a negative energy balance, or burn more calories than they take in, to reduce their weight. Increased physical activity can be beneficial, but diet is also crucial. The kinds and amounts of food consumed can significantly affect caloric intake and, thus, the results of weight loss.

The Macronutrients

The macronutrients that makeup nutrition—fats, proteins, and carbohydrates—all have distinct functions in the body.

1. *Carbohydrates:* The body uses carbohydrates as its primary energy source. But not every carbohydrate is made equally.

Whole grains, fruits, and vegetables are examples of complex carbohydrates that provide essential nutrients and fiber, aiding in digestion and increasing feelings of fullness. Simple carbohydrates, which are present in processed foods and sugary snacks, can raise blood sugar levels quickly and boost appetite, making it hard to maintain a calorie deficit.

2. **_Proteins:_** Proteins are necessary for the growth and maintenance of tissues, especially muscle. Eating enough protein can help you retain muscle mass while reducing weight because muscle burns more calories than fat. Lean meats, beans, lentils, and dairy products are examples of high-protein diets that promote satiety, which helps regulate appetite and cut calories.

3. **_Fats:_** Healthy fats found in avocados, almonds, and olive oil are essential for the synthesis of hormones, the absorption of nutrients, and the health of the brain. Although dietary fat has a lot of calories, it can also make you feel full, which makes it simpler to follow a diet that limits calories. Portion sizes must be carefully considered, though, as too much fat can lead to a rise in caloric intake.

To create a well-rounded diet that encourages weight loss, it is essential to comprehend the ratios of these macronutrients. Focusing on complete, minimally processed foods that offer a range of nutrients while controlling calorie consumption is a common tactic.

The Value of Portion Management

Portion control is crucial for weight loss even while eating nutrient-dense foods. A lot of people overeat because they underestimate portion sizes. People can become more conscious of their portion sizes by practicing mindful eating, which involves observing their hunger and fullness cues.

How to effectively manage portions:

- ❖ Use Smaller Plates: This simple strategy can help you reduce the likelihood of overeating by limiting serving sizes.
- ❖ Examine nutrition labels: Being aware of an item's calorie count and serving size can assist consumers in making wise choices.
- ❖ Pre-portion Snacks: You can avoid mindless snacking right out of the packet by preparing individual snacks in advance.

Fiber's Contribution to Weight Loss

Dietary fiber is essential for weight loss because it facilitates digestion and increases feelings of fullness. It can be found in fruits, vegetables, whole grains, and legumes. Because high-fiber foods take longer to chew and digest, you are less likely to overeat and feel satiated for longer.

Fiber supports beneficial gut flora, which may have an impact on weight control and metabolism. Including a range of foods high in fiber in your diet not only aids in weight loss but also enhances your general health and well-being.

Hydration and Loss of Weight

When talking about losing weight, it's easy to forget to drink enough water. Digestion and metabolism are two of the many bodily functions that depend on water. Hunger and thirst can be mistaken for one another, leading to unnecessary snacking. People can reduce their calorie intake and feel fuller by drinking water before meals.

Herbal teas and other low-calorie drinks can help you stay hydrated without consuming additional calories, in addition to water. Consuming sugary drinks should be done with caution because they have no nutritional value and can quickly result in calorie excess.

Reducing weight has psychological ramifications in addition to physical ones. Weight loss attempts might be hampered by stress, emotional eating, and food-related behaviors. Building good coping techniques may be facilitated by an understanding of the emotional factors that contribute to overeating. You can manage these problems with the aid of professional assistance, stress-reduction techniques, and mindfulness.

In summary, diet has a key role in weight loss by controlling metabolism, energy balance, and overall health. By understanding the significance of macronutrients, practicing portion control, giving fiber and water priority, and creating sustainable meal plans, people can help themselves achieve their weight loss goals. Additionally, by comprehending the psychological aspects of eating, you can create a more positive relationship with food, which will make it easier to achieve and sustain weight loss over time. Following these guidelines encourages a better, more balanced lifestyle in addition to weight loss.

How To Create An Eco-Friendly Meal Plan

Creating a sustainable diet plan is essential for long-term health and weight loss. In addition to assisting you in making food choices, a well-organized meal plan ensures that your meals are wholesome, balanced, and consistent with your health objectives. In order to make sure they fit into your long-term lifestyle, we'll break down the essential elements of developing a sustainable meal plan into manageable steps below.

1. Recognize your dietary requirements

Understanding your unique dietary demands is essential when creating a meal plan. Age, gender, degree of activity, and health goals can all affect these. Maintaining a macronutrient balance—proteins, fats, and carbohydrates—while avoiding severely restricting any one food type is crucial while trying to reduce weight.

❖ Calories: For gradual, healthy weight loss, a moderate calorie deficit—roughly 500 fewer calories per day than your maintenance level—is typically advised.

❖ Macronutrients: Aim for a meal that has roughly 40% carbs, 30% protein, and 30% good fats. Although you can adjust this ratio to suit your needs, this well-rounded approach encourages weight loss without depriving your body of essential nutrients.

For instance:

Your meal plan can consist of the following to reach a daily calorie consumption of 1,500:

60% of the 600 calories came from carbs.

30% of the 450 calories come from protein.

30% of the 450 calories come from fat.

2. Arrange a variety of well-balanced meals

Adding diversity to your meals is one of the keys to sustainability. Consuming the same foods every day could become boring and lead to fatigue and desires. Plan meals that are easy to prepare and contain a range of veggies, proteins, and nutritious grains to prevent this.

❖ Proteins: Consume lean proteins such as lentils, fish, poultry, turkey, and tofu. These will help you feel fuller for longer and keep your muscular mass.

❖ Vegetables: Aim to have different colored vegetables on half of your plate. This guarantees a varied spectrum of vitamins, minerals, and antioxidants in addition to adding diversity. Both fresh and cooked vegetables can provide different flavors and textures to your food.

❖ Whole Grains and Fiber: Whole grains that aid in digestion, such as brown rice, quinoa, and whole-wheat bread, are rich in fiber. Additionally, fiber helps you feel full and prevents overeating.

An example of a daily meal plan:

Breakfast consists of an omelet loaded with spinach, tomatoes, and mushrooms, accompanied with avocado and whole wheat toast.

Lunch consists of quinoa, mixed greens, grilled chicken salad, and a mild vinaigrette.

Brown rice, roasted broccoli, carrots, zucchini, and baked fish are served for supper.

3. Portion control

One of the best ways to create a long-term meal plan is to learn how to control portion sizes. The amount of food we consume has a greater impact on weight loss than the type of food we consume. Calculating calories at each meal is not necessary, although it is helpful to be aware of amounts.

❖ Protein Portions: A protein portion should be about the size of your hand.
❖ Carbohydrate Portions: A portion of carbohydrates, like rice or pasta, should be around the size of your fist.

❖ Vegetables: You can eat a lot of vegetables without worrying about portion sizes because they are high in fiber and low in calories. Just make sure they aren't slathered with oil or butter.

❖ Fats: Moderate consumption is advised for healthy fats found in nuts, seeds, and oils. Every meal should contain around a thumb's worth of good fats.

Portion control is just being more aware of how much food you need to be satisfied; it does not involve deprivation.

4. Include batch cooking and meal preparation

Maintaining a sustainable meal plan requires consistency, and planning meals is one of the simplest ways to do it. The practice of preparing some or all of your meals in advance, known as meal prep, makes It simpler to stick to your schedule, even on busy days.

❖ To prepare larger quantities of cereals, meats, and vegetables, schedule time once or twice a week. These can be stored in portioned containers for convenient and rapid assembly throughout the week.

❖ Some dishes, like casseroles, stews, and soups, can be frozen for later use. This is particularly helpful when you want a healthy, prepared dinner but don't feel like cooking.

❖ In addition to saving time, meal planning prevents you from choosing poor meals on the spur of the moment because of a lack of energy or time.

5. Be flexible

A sustainable diet plan needs to be both well-organized and adaptable. Your timetable will occasionally be interrupted since life is unpredictable. Your meal plan should be viewed as a guide rather than a strict framework. Being flexible allows you to adjust as necessary without feeling like a failure.

❖ When dining out, go for healthier options like salads, grilled proteins, or dishes made with vegetables. Never be afraid to ask for changes, like veggies in place of fries or dressing on the side.

❖ It's acceptable and beneficial for long-term success to occasionally indulge in your favorite foods. Giving yourself a treat occasionally helps to avoid feelings of deprivation and curb cravings, both of which can result in overeating.

Finding balance and enjoying food while maintaining your goals is the aim of a sustainable plan, not perfection.

6. Pay attention to your body

Creating a sustainable food plan requires you to learn to listen to your body. This entails recognizing the difference between emotional eating and true hunger, eating when you are hungry, and stopping when you are full.

❖ Try eating mindfully by avoiding distractions like TV and cell phones. This helps you prevent overeating by making you more conscious of when you're full.
❖ Pay attention to your body's signals. Are you bored, anxious, or upset, or are you hungry? You can prevent overeating by being aware of these signs.

You may improve your health and well-being by cultivating a positive relationship with food through mindful eating.

7. Monitor your development and adapt as necessary

You may make your food plan more sustainable by regularly reviewing your progress and strategy. The objective is to be aware of your progress, so it doesn't have to be hard to track. You can use a smartphone app, log your meals, or just keep track of how your clothes fit.

Your nutritional needs will evolve along with your body. Try changing your portion sizes, eating more vegetables, or getting more exercise if you hit a stall in your weight loss efforts.

A sustainable eating plan is a long-term lifestyle shift rather than a quick fix. You can ensure that your food plan keeps supporting your goals over time by being flexible and often assessing your progress.

Lastly, creating a sustainable meal plan requires a blend of mindful eating, flexibility, and meticulous preparation. By including a variety of nutrient-dense foods, controlling portion sizes, and preparing meals in advance, you can succeed over the long run. Enjoy the journey to better health, pay attention to your body, and modify as necessary.

Easy Meal Planning Techniques For Active Lives

One of the best strategies to keep up a healthy diet, particularly if you're trying to reduce weight, is to schedule your meals. Convenience foods, such as takeout, are simple to reach for when you're pressed for time and are frequently higher in calories and less nutritious. But without spending hours in the kitchen, you may provide your body with wholesome meals that aid in weight loss with a little planning and preparation. Here are some simple, doable tips to help you stay on course even with a busy schedule.

1. Make a weekly plan first

Having a well-defined plan is essential to effective meal planning. Make time to organize your meals at the start of every week. This process doesn't have to be difficult or time-consuming. Writing down what you eat over the following five or seven days is a good place to start. Make sure that every meal—breakfast, lunch, supper, and snacks—is nutritionally balanced.

Eat meals that are moderately rich in carbohydrates and high in lean protein, fiber, and healthy fats if you want to lose weight. To organize this, simply see your plate as having half of veggies, a quarter of lean protein (such as fish, poultry, tofu, or lentils), and the remaining quarter of whole grains or complex carbohydrates.

2. For efficiency, cook in batches

Making a fresh meal every day can be daunting when you're pressed for time. Cooking in batches is a useful strategy. On the weekend or any other day when you have some free time, dedicate a few hours to cooking larger amounts of food that can be utilized for several meals. This can entail making a big pot of soup or stew, roasting vegetables, or grilling some chicken breasts. After the meals are prepared, store them in separate containers for convenient grab-and-go throughout the week.

Because you are less likely to choose unhealthy, last-minute food options when you have wholesome meals on hand, batch cooking also helps you stay on track with your nutrition goals.

3. Getting the ingredients ready beforehand

If you are not comfortable preparing entire meals in advance, consider preparing items in advance. During a busy workday, this tactic helps you maintain diversity while saving time. Take the time to chop vegetables, cook grains like brown rice or quinoa, and prepare lean proteins like sautéed tofu or baked chicken so that you just need to reheat and assemble your meal when it's time to cook.

Basic elements that can be used in many different cuisines can also be made. Roasted sweet potatoes, for instance, work well in salads, as a side dish, or even in breakfast scrambles. You may use cooked chicken in stir-fries, salads, and wraps.

4. Make use of healthy and adaptable staples

Keep wholesome essentials in your kitchen that you can quickly mix and match to create a range of meals. Lean meats (chicken, fish, eggs, or plant-based proteins), canned beans, frozen vegetables, and wholesome cereals are all readily available and easy to prepare. These ingredients can be added to salads, stir-fries, and soups, among other recipes.

You can resist the urge to order takeout or reach for processed food when you're hungry and pressed for time by always keeping wholesome necessities on hand.

5. Make use of freezing power

A great approach to save time and guarantee that you always have wholesome options on hand is to freeze meals. Many foods retain their flavor and nutritional value when frozen and reheated. Examples include casseroles, stews, soups, and even whole-grain pancakes or muffins.

Freeze individual portions for later use when cooking larger quantities. To make it easier to locate what you need, mark containers with the date and contents. Even on the busiest days, you can maintain your meal plan by keeping a selection of pre-cooked meals in the freezer.

6. Make easy and quick recipes a priority

Recipes that take little time or effort to prepare are a good choice when meal planning for a busy lifestyle. Seek out recipes that are easy to prepare and call for a few ingredients. For instance, because they require less active cooking time, slow cooker recipes, one-pot meals, and sheet pan dinners are great options.

Think of preparing dishes like grain bowls, protein-rich salads, or stir-fries that can be prepared in less than 30 minutes. These dinners are flexible and stress-free since they can be customized to use whatever ingredients you have on hand.

7. Make provisions for leftovers

For people who are constantly on the go, leftovers are their best friend. Make extra pieces of your dinner so you can eat lunch or dinner the next day. This guarantees that you have a healthy dinner without having to prepare anything extra, in addition to saving time.

For instance, if you're grilling chicken and veggies for dinner, prepare extra and eat the leftovers for lunch the following day in a salad or wrap. Additionally, leftovers can be frozen for later use.

8. Simple snacks are ideal

Any weight-loss plan should include healthy snacks, particularly if you're pressed for time. Snacks should be straightforward and high in nutrients. Here are some easy choices:

- Hummus and sliced veggies
- Berries, bananas, and apples are examples of fresh fruit.
- Mixed seeds or nuts.
- Honey-drizzled Greek yogurt.
- Crackers are made with whole grains and almond butter.

Having nutritious snacks on hand reduces the temptation to eat processed or sugary foods when you're hungry. These snacks are also portable, easy to prepare, and provide long-lasting energy in between meals.

9. Make use of tools and technology

Utilize technology to make meal planning easier: Several meal planning apps can assist you with organizing your weekly meals, making grocery lists, and suggesting recipes based on your dietary preferences. Appliances such as air fryers, slow cookers, and instant pots help make meals quickly and with minimal supervision.

In the same way that an air fryer enables you to cook crispy vegetables or lean proteins more quickly and with less oil than traditional frying methods, a slow cooker, for instance, enables you to combine ingredients in the morning and have a fully cooked meal by dinnertime without any effort.

10. Remain adaptable and allow for improvisation

A few "emergency" healthy meals or snacks, like a quick salad, a freezer meal you've already prepared, or a simple stir-fry with premade components, should be on hand. While meal preparation is the key to staying on track, flexibility is also necessary and sometimes life gets in the way.

You can adjust your plan in response to cravings or last-minute plans without feeling confined if you give yourself some leeway.

Organizing, planning, and making the most of your time are all crucial, and with a little practice, meal planning may become second nature, enabling you to maintain a healthy diet no matter how busy your schedule gets. Meal planning does not have to be difficult or time-consuming, and even if you lead a busy lifestyle, you can prepare healthy, balanced meals that can aid in weight loss.

CHAPTER 7: MAINTAINING MOTIVATION AND MONITORING DEVELOPMENT

Recognizing The Benefits Of Maintaining Consistency In Your Practice

The idea of consistency shows up as a crucial element for success while pursuing health and wellness objectives, especially weight loss and improved mobility. Major and lasting changes can result from maintaining a consistent practice, whether it be chair yoga or another type of exercise. The significance of consistency, the physical and mental benefits, and helpful advice for forming a regular chair yoga practice are all covered in this essay.

The Influence of Habit Development

Consistency and the psychology of habit formation are closely intertwined. Doing something regularly helps you keep to it over time since it becomes a part of your daily or weekly routine. A study found that depending on the activity's intricacy and the personality of the person, developing a new habit might take anywhere from 21 to 66 days. Because chair yoga may be done in a comfortable setting without the need for specific equipment, it can be an accessible beginning point for many people, especially the elderly and those with limited mobility.

Chair yoga turns from a chore to a habit as it becomes a part of your everyday routine. This shift is crucial since habits require less willpower and mental effort to sustain, freeing you up to focus on other aspects of your life. By prioritizing chair yoga on your calendar, you are committing to a whole lifestyle change that fosters mindfulness, relaxation, and a closer relationship with your body in addition to physical fitness.

Gaining Flexibility and Strength Over Time

A noticeable benefit of regular chair yoga practice is a gradual improvement in strength and flexibility. Chair yoga emphasizes serene, controlled movements that are kinder to the body than high-intensity exercises, which may yield quick benefits but can also be harmful. Strength and flexibility are enhanced as a result of muscles and joints adapting via regular practice.

The elderly greatly benefit from this element. Many elderly people lose muscle mass and flexibility, which increases their risk of falls and accidents. Regular chair yoga practice can help seniors avoid these negative effects by enhancing their ability to perform daily tasks, preserving their balance, and reducing their risk of injury.

Muscle memory is also aided by consistent practice. Your body becomes more acclimated to certain postures and motions as you practice them, which eventually leads to improved form and efficacy. This is particularly crucial for new yoga practitioners because learning the right posture and technique can improve results and make the practice more pleasurable.

Benefits to the Mind and Emotion

In addition to the physical advantages, consistent practice has an effect on mental and emotional health. Regular chair yoga practice has been linked to lower levels of anxiety, sadness, and stress. The calming effects of yoga, combined with an emphasis on mindfulness and breathing, promote mental clarity and emotional healing.

You may foster a self-care environment by committing to a regular practice. You can unwind, think, and re-establish a connection with your thoughts and feelings by taking this time for yourself. Being more conscious of your body and thoughts might result in a feeling of empowerment. Regular chair yoga can provide you with positive reinforcement that can increase your self-esteem and encourage you to experiment with other healthy habits, such as improving your diet and social interactions.

Getting Past Consistency Obstacles

Maintaining a regular chair yoga practice can be challenging, despite the clear advantages of consistency. Potential obstacles include physical restrictions, time limits, and periods of low motivation. But understanding these challenges and coming up with strategies to get beyond them can make all the difference.

❖ Set Achievable Objectives: To start, decide on realistic objectives for your chair yoga practice. Try starting with 15 to 20 minutes a few times a week rather than trying to complete an hour-long workout every day. As you become more accustomed to and comfortable with your habit, gradually increase the frequency and length.

❖ Plan Your Practice: Consider chair yoga classes to be important appointments. Set up time on your schedule, just like you would for a social gathering or a visit to the doctor. Routine is the foundation of consistency, so scheduling practice time could help foster this habit.

❖ Establish a Supportive Environment: Choose a comfortable and tranquil space for your practice. Limit distractions, provide enough illumination, and pick a cozy chair. Surround oneself with inspiring objects, such as words of wisdom or images, to create a positive atmosphere.

❖ Buddy Up: Invite a loved one to attend chair yoga sessions with you. In addition to providing accountability, practicing with a partner can boost motivation and make the activity more pleasurable. Creating a supportive group can also be facilitated by sharing your struggles and accomplishments.

❖ Monitor Your Progress: You can maintain your motivation and attention by keeping a journal or log of your practice. Note the date, the length of each session, and any feelings or insights that come up. Your commitment to consistency may be strengthened by minor successes.

❖ Be Adaptable: Maintaining flexibility is just as vital as consistency. Because life can be unexpected, you might not be able to train as regularly on some days. Rather than giving up, find innovative ways to include chair yoga into your everyday schedule. This can be practicing breathing techniques before bedtime or performing a few easy stretches while watching television.

The Consistent Ripple Effect

There are numerous benefits to practicing chair yoga consistently. You can improve other areas of your life by practicing yoga, which can help you develop discipline and mindfulness. Increased energy levels brought on by improved physical health often enable you to engage more fully in daily tasks, hobbies, and social gatherings. While increased resilience can make it easier for you to handle life's challenges, improved mental clarity can help you solve difficulties and make better judgments.

Additionally, as your chair yoga practice progresses, you could encourage people around you to put their health and well-being first. By sharing your successes, setbacks, and experiences, you may encourage and assist others as they set out on their fitness journeys.

For chair yoga and overall wellbeing to be successful, consistency is essential. You can reap the physical, mental, and emotional rewards of making time for your health by establishing a regular practice. You will probably find that small, gradual changes over time result in significant changes as you embrace the journey of consistency, enhancing your quality of life and promoting a long-term, healthy lifestyle. Keep in mind that the path to well-being is a marathon rather than a sprint;

embrace the process and allow consistency to lead you to your objectives.

Establishing Reasonable Objectives For Flexibility And Weight Loss

Setting reasonable and attainable goals is one of the most crucial steps in any fitness or weight loss program. It's simple to be swept up in the excitement of change and set unrealistic or overly ambitious goals, which might lead to weariness, injury, or discontent. Setting specific, measurable, and achievable goals is essential when incorporating chair yoga into your practice, particularly if your objectives include weight loss and increased flexibility. This will keep you motivated and on track.

You must first evaluate your current level of fitness and physical limitations before setting any goals. Although everyone is different, chair yoga is a low-impact, easily accessible form of exercise that is suitable for people of all fitness levels. Some people may start with significant mobility issues, while others may be physically fit but wish to improve their flexibility or shed a few pounds.

You must honestly assess your current circumstances before setting any feasible ambitions. This can be achieved by taking into account:

❖ Your Current Weight: To track your development, find your starting weight. But don't only pay attention to the scale's number. Weight loss is erratic, and strength training-induced muscle growth can sometimes offset weight loss.

❖ Mobility and flexibility: Assess your existing range of motion. Are you able to feel your toes? How simple is it for you to get up from a seated posture, bend, or twist? This will assist you in setting a starting point for your flexibility objectives.

❖ Strength and Endurance: How long can you maintain the fundamental chair yoga poses? Is it possible to finish a sequence without getting tired? With the help of these indicators, you can set little objectives to build strength and stamina.

Knowing where you're coming from enables you to tailor your objectives to your unique needs and skills, making them more doable and practical.

Establishing SMART objectives

Goals that follow the SMART framework—Specific, Measurable, Achievable, Relevant, and Timebound—are the most successful. Let's examine how this idea relates to goals for flexibility and weight loss.

❖ Specific: Be as clear as you can about your objectives. Saying "I want to lose weight" is not as effective as saying "I want to improve my eating habits and do chair yoga three times a week." Similarly, saying "I want to become more flexible" is not as effective as saying "I want to increase my ability to touch my toes within 30 days of daily practice."

❖ Measurable: You need to have a way to track your progress. Weekly weigh-ins, measures of inches lost, or progress pictures could be examples of this. To increase your flexibility, note how far you can extend in each stance. Test your hands' range of motion during a forward bend or your torso's ease of twisting, for instance.

❖ Achievable: Your objectives ought to be demanding but doable. Most people can't get completely flexible overnight or lose thirty pounds in a month, especially when starting a new workout regimen like chair yoga. You will succeed if you set tiny, achievable goals, like losing 1-2 pounds a week or progressively improving your flexibility over a few months.

❖ Relevant: Your objectives have to align with your overarching well-being goals. Your objectives should center on activities and routines that support weight loss and flexibility if those are your main concerns. Examples of these are regular chair yoga, food tracking, and exercises that improve flexibility. Don't set objectives that are too distant from these important regions.

❖ Time-bound: To establish focus and a sense of urgency, set a deadline for your goals. Establish goals that are both short- and long-term, such as "I want to lose 5 pounds in the next month" or "I want to be able to perform a full chair sun salutation sequence without stopping within six weeks." Having deadlines keeps you motivated and lets you celebrate your accomplishments when you hit each goal.

Goals for Flexibility and Weight Loss Should Be Balanced

It is important to keep in mind that although flexibility and weight loss can work in tandem, they are two distinct objectives that may progress at different rates. By burning calories, raising your metabolism, and reducing stress, chair yoga, which emphasizes breathing, stretching, and strengthening, can help you lose weight. If you want to lose weight, you must be patient because chair yoga cannot burn as many calories as more strenuous exercises.

At the same time, flexibility can be increased in small or large steps. You might discover that you can twist a little bit more in a sitting spinal twist one week and that you can bend much more deeply in a seated forward fold the next week. Since increases in flexibility might be small and gradual, it's important to design goals that account for this steady but modest growth.

Think about establishing two objectives to balance both, like aiming to lose a specified amount of weight and mastering a particular yoga posture over a predetermined amount of time. For instance, in the next four weeks, you could aim to lose five pounds and increase your range of motion in a seated pigeon stance. In this manner, you can concentrate on multiple aspects of your health journey instead of just one outcome.

Creating a program that encourages both weight loss and increased flexibility is essential when setting goals. Chair yoga involves planning a well-rounded weekly schedule that includes breathing techniques to enhance overall wellness, stretches to improve flexibility and strength-building poses.

Here is an example of a weekly routine:
- Monday: Stretching and flexibility-focused chair yoga.
- Wednesday: Strengthening and toning chair yoga exercises, such as chair squats and seated leg raises.
- Friday: A thorough chair yoga course that blends strength and flexibility exercises.
- Sunday: A stress-relieving, weight-loss-promoting meditation and deep breathing session.

Your chances of remaining engaged and improving are increased when you vary your regimen. Losing weight and increasing flexibility requires consistent practice.

Setting reasonable chair yoga weight loss and flexibility goals necessitates knowing where you are coming from, creating clear, achievable objectives, and striking a balance between the mental and physical aspects of the journey. You'll find yourself gradually advancing toward your fitness objectives if you have perseverance, resolve, and a laser-like focus.

Keeping A Progress Journal With Milestones, Measurements, And Pictures

One of the best ways to stay motivated and monitor your progress toward improved mobility, weight loss, and overall health with chair yoga is to keep a progress journal. It allows you to record concrete proof of your development, evaluate your achievements, and stay true to your goals. You can create a customized road map to your goals and discover what suits your body and lifestyle by recording measurements, taking pictures, and setting milestones.

Many individuals just take the scale's reading into account when it comes to improving their mobility and losing weight. Although weight is an important parameter, performance can be measured in other ways as well. It might be annoying at times to rely solely on your weight, particularly if you have plateaus or slight fluctuations brought on by water retention, muscle growth, or normal body cycles. A comprehensive progress journal can help with this.

You can gain a more comprehensive understanding of your development by monitoring many indicators, including body measurements, flexibility levels, photos, and fitness milestones. You may identify non-scale achievements like improved strength, flexibility, or the ability to perform increasingly difficult chair yoga poses thanks to this multidimensional tracking. Additionally, it encourages consistency and maintains your attention on your task, both of which are critical for long-term success.

Measuring and Recording

When doing chair yoga to lose weight, measurements are a crucial part of monitoring results. Measures offer a more reliable and consistent picture of changes in body composition, even if weight varies daily and does not always correspond to changes in muscle tone or fat loss. You could want to monitor your arms, chest, hips, thighs, waist, and any other trouble spots where you'd like to see more definition or fat loss.

Here's how to take and document measurements accurately:

❖ Measure the narrowest part of your waist, which is typically just above the belly button, using a flexible measuring tape. Keep the tape level around your body and make sure it is snug but not too tight.
❖ Measure the widest point of your hips, which is usually around your glutes, while standing with your feet together. Verify that the tape is straight and level around your body.

❖ Take consistent measures of the widest part of each thigh, as these may differ from leg to leg.
❖ Measure the bicep about the midpoint of the elbow and shoulder, ideally on your dominant arm.
❖ Using taut but not restrictive tape, measure around the largest part of your chest.

To assess how your body changes over time, it is helpful to take these measurements at regular intervals, like once a month or every two weeks. For future reference, record your measurements in a progress notebook and date them.

The Influence of Photography

Recording progress photos is a terrific way to visually document your chair yoga journey in addition to recording measurements. When you look in the mirror every day, it's easy to overlook small gains because physical changes might happen gradually. Progress pictures provide a clear visual depiction of your body's changes over time and can be quite inspiring, particularly when the scale's readings don't fully capture the situation.

Here are some tips for taking progress photographs that work:

1. Opt for a well-fitting attire that highlights your body type, like form-fitting athletic wear. Wear the same attire for every round of shots to ensure consistency.

2. Take pictures in the same spot every time, preferably in a well-lit area or with natural light. A simple background makes the changes in your body stand out.

3. To obtain a complete view of how your body is evolving, take pictures of your development from the front, side, and rear. This will provide you with a more comprehensive view of your changes.

4. It's recommended to take pictures every two to four weeks, just like with measurements. As you see tangible results of your efforts, you will be able to compare your progress and stay motivated.

5. Print your progress images and store them in your progress notebook, or store them in a folder on your computer or phone. Comparing these pictures can be a potent way to remind yourself of how far you've come, particularly on days when progress seems to be sluggish.

Establishing Benchmarks

Milestones are particular achievements that act as benchmarks for your chair yoga journey. They provide you with clear objectives to strive for and a milestone to commemorate along the road. It's crucial to incorporate a range of realistic, reachable, and personally meaningful short- and long-term goals while setting milestones.

Here's how to create milestones that work:

1. Short-term milestones: These are more immediate, smaller objectives that will help you stay motivated and focused. Finishing your first full week of chair yoga, mastering a particular pose, like the Seated Forward Bend, or losing your first inch around your waist are examples of short-term goals.

2. Long-term milestones: These are more ambitious objectives that will require more time to accomplish but show significant advancement. Examples include reaching a particular degree of flexibility, losing a particular amount of weight, or executing increasingly difficult poses like Seated Boat Pose or Chair Warrior III.

3. Non-scale milestones: Keep in mind to create objectives that go beyond simply losing weight. For instance, you may incorporate additional breathing techniques into your routine to reduce tension, concentrate on enhancing your balance, or increase your stamina during chair yoga sessions.

4. Reward yourself: It's important to celebrate when you accomplish a goal! This means rewarding yourself in ways that advance your objective, not indulging in unhealthy habits. Buy a new yoga mat, have a massage, or arrange a relaxing activity to honor your diligence and hard work.

Holding yourself accountable is one of the main benefits of maintaining a progress journal. You're moving forward in your journey when you record your measurements, write down how you feel after each workout or comment on what's been working. You can identify trends and make adjustments if something isn't functioning as planned with the help of a progress record.

Every week, set aside some time to consider your physical and mental well-being. Are you feeling more resilient? More adaptable? Is your vitality increasing? Together with the tangible proof of measurements and photos, these reflections provide a potent story of change.

You may monitor physical changes in your body and strengthen your commitment to your health and well-being by regularly documenting and evaluating your progress. Maintaining a progress journal during your chair yoga journey will help you stay motivated, regardless of your goals—whether they be weight loss, mobility restoration, or just improving your quality of life.

Getting Past Setbacks and Remaining Devoted

Every fitness or weight loss journey eventually reaches a plateau. Despite your best efforts, it can be disheartening when the progress you've worked so hard to achieve seems to stall. Although plateaus might be depressing, they can also present chances for development, education, and reorientation. Plateaus are a natural part of the body's adaptation process. It takes a combination of dietary, mental, and physical changes to break through weight reduction plateaus in chair yoga. Maintaining your commitment at this stage is essential to achieving your goals and long-term success.

When the body no longer reacts to the same diet or exercise regimen that used to produce results, a plateau occurs. Muscle memory, the body becoming more adept at burning calories, and even changes in metabolism as you lose weight are some of the reasons why this can happen. After the initial excitement and advancement of a new training regimen, when the body has had an opportunity to adapt, plateaus are particularly common.

As with any fitness regimen, your body will eventually adapt to chair yoga poses. With time, the same tasks that were challenging at first could get easier, resulting in reduced energy loss with each session. This is a key factor that could cause weight loss to stall or even reverse.

By realizing that plateaus are a typical part of the process, you may be able to go from frustration to inspiration. Consider a plateau as an opportunity to make adjustments and challenge your body in new ways rather than as a setback.

Techniques for Breaking Through Plateaus

1. Make your chair yoga practice more varied

One of the best ways to overcome a plateau in your fitness is to switch up your routine. This can be doing additional repetitions of particular poses, stepping up the intensity of your practice, or embracing new positions in chair yoga.

For instance, try adding more dynamic workouts like Chair Push-ups or Seated Bicycle Crunches to your routine of basic stances like Chair Warrior or Seated Mountain. These postures increase cardiovascular challenge and target a variety of muscle groups, which increases calorie expenditure.

Additionally, by switching up the sequence in which you perform the poses, you keep your body curious and avoid habituation. Your workouts can be made even more challenging by incorporating more difficult poses like Chair Reverse Plank and Seated Eagle Pose, which will raise your metabolism and re-engage your muscles.

2. Gradually increase the intensity

Increase the intensity of your chair yoga exercises gradually if you want to continue seeing results. This does not necessarily mean making big changes, but over time, small, steady improvements can make a big difference.

Hold positions for extended lengths of time, add resistance (such as resistance bands or light weights), or accelerate your transitions between poses to up the ante. For instance, your leg and core muscles may be strained if you hold the Seated Chair Squat for a further 10 to 15 seconds. Similar to this, increasing muscular engagement during seated leg lifts or seated hamstring stretches with resistance bands will promote fat loss and muscle growth.

3. Increase the number of cardiovascular exercises

Strength, flexibility, and balance are the main goals of chair yoga, but adding more cardiovascular movements could help you burn more calories and get beyond plateaus. Chair-based aerobic exercises that increase heart rate and intensity include chair jumping jacks, sat marching, and sitting toe taps.

In addition to your usual chair yoga regimen, even brief bursts of activity can make a big difference. To keep your body active and avoid adaptation, think about switching between quick bursts of aerobic and strength-focused positions.

4. Pay attention to healthy eating

Although chair yoga is an excellent method for weight loss, reaching weight loss plateaus also needs a proper diet. When the body does not receive the right nutritional balance to support ongoing improvement, weight reduction may stall.

Make sure your diet supports your weight loss objectives by emphasizing complex carbohydrates, lean proteins, healthy fats, and whole foods. Steer clear of processed foods, added sugars, and bad fats as they might slow down your metabolism and cause plateaus.

Consider including more high-protein meals in your diet if it is lacking because protein helps build and repair muscles, which can increase your metabolism. In a similar vein, it's critical to drink lots of water because dehydration might hinder your metabolism. Additionally, try to keep your portion sizes to a minimum because, if overindulged, even healthy meals can help you maintain your weight.

5. Recuperation and rest

When the body has been overworked and has not had enough time to recover, a plateau may form. Your progress may stall if you've been exerting yourself too much because your muscles may grow tired.

In between workouts, give your body enough time to recuperate. This doesn't mean you have to stop doing chair yoga entirely; instead, think about including more calming methods like breathing exercises, meditation, or gentle stretching. These can help reduce stress, improve muscle repair, and provide your body with new energy for future exercises.

Keep in mind that relaxation is a crucial component of the fitness and weight-loss process. Ironically, overtraining can lead to injury, burnout, and a growth stall.

Staying Devoted Throughout Plateaus

It can be challenging to stay committed during a plateau since dissatisfaction might arise from not seeing any progress. To overcome this brief phase and achieve long-term success, however, dedication is necessary.

1. **Monitor victories that are not scaled:** If the scale's number isn't changing, check for additional growth indicators. These "non-scale victories" could be improved balance, flexibility, endurance, or even stress reduction. If the scale doesn't inspire you, you can be inspired by the way your body feels, the ease with which you can perform specific poses or even the way your clothes fit.

2. **Establish fresh, attainable objectives:** A plateau offers a chance to establish fresh, immediate objectives. These can be more focused on building your strength, perfecting a particular chair yoga pose, or extending your practice time than they are on weight loss. By shifting your focus from weight reduction to other areas of exercise, you might rekindle your motivation.

3. **Remain patient and upbeat:** It takes perseverance and a good outlook to break through a plateau. Keep in mind that losing weight is not a straight line, and it could take some time for the body to adapt before showing signs of improvement. Remind yourself frequently of why you embarked on this journey in the first place and keep a good outlook. Honor small victories while remembering your long-term objectives.

4. **Look for accountability and support:** Maintaining commitment during challenging times can be greatly impacted by having a support network. It might be supportive to share your struggles and experiences with a friend, relative, or online community. To hold yourself accountable, track your progress, and recognize your achievements along the road, you can also use tools like progress journals or apps.

It takes a combination of strategy, perseverance, and self-awareness to break through plateaus and stay dedicated. You can overcome the plateau and keep going toward your objectives by switching up your chair yoga routine, progressively increasing the level of difficulty, eating healthily, and emphasizing relaxation and recuperation. Above all, keep in mind that plateaus are just temporary and that long-term success will eventually result from remaining dedicated to your objective.

CONCLUSION

As we draw to a close our exploration of this volume, it's critical to consider the fundamental concepts that have brought you this far. Through the gentle yet effective practice of chair yoga, this book aims to provide you with the skills, information, and inspiration you need to go on a transformative path of weight loss, improved mobility, and enhanced flexibility.

We've examined in the chapters how chair yoga offers a holistic approach to health and wellbeing, going beyond simply being a form of exercise. People of various ages, skill levels, and fitness levels can engage in chair yoga, a sustainable form of exercise that takes little time or effort yet has enormous health benefits. It integrates the breath, body, and mind to support internal healing and harmony.

You gain more than just the physical benefits of improved strength, flexibility, and mobility when you integrate movement, breathing, and mindfulness. You've also realized that chair yoga can help you feel better emotionally and mentally. By lowering tension, improving focus, and fostering a sense of serenity, chair yoga helps with many of the emotional problems that commonly accompany weight loss efforts.

The importance of consistency in your chair yoga practice is the book's main lesson. For long-term weight loss and physical improvement, commitment is necessary. You now know that even small, everyday routines, like breathing techniques or simple sitting positions, can have a significant impact on your physical and emotional well-being over time.

From beginner to intermediate, the activities in the book are designed to progress alongside you. You have a strategy for success, regardless of whether you're just starting or wish to advance your profession. Being consistent just means showing up for yourself, whether you have five minutes or thirty. It does not entail perfection. Any journey will inevitably encounter setbacks, but resiliency and getting back to your practice can help you stay on course to meet your objectives.

One of the main tenets of chair yoga is breathwork, which has been highlighted as a powerful method for stress relief, raising metabolism, and improving digestion. You have studied several breathing techniques that can aid in weight loss, such as box breathing, diaphragmatic breathing, and alternate nostril breathing. These exercises help to increase brain clarity, control hunger, and soothe the nervous system.

Both on and off the yoga chair, incorporating these breathing techniques into your daily practice can make a big difference.

You may stay focused on your wellness objectives, prevent emotional eating, and lower anxiety by practicing deep, mindful breathing.

You have also read about the significance of diet for both weight loss and general health in this book. A healthy diet enhances your chair yoga practice by giving your body the nutrients it needs to burn fat, gain strength, and recover from exercise.

The idea of mindful eating, which has its roots in yogic philosophy, aids in the development of a healthy relationship with food. When combined with mindful eating practices, chair yoga helps you pay attention to your body's hunger signals, savor your meals with awareness, and prevent overindulging. This method helps you lose weight and achieve emotional balance with food, as you have seen in earlier chapters.

Physical transformation and weight loss are nonlinear processes, and obstacles are normal along the route. The adaptability of chair yoga is among its most significant features. You can still perform simple movements or concentrate on breathing techniques on days when you're feeling emotionally or physically worn out. You can do chair yoga at any point in your wellness journey.

Enjoying small victories, such as losing a few pounds, increasing your range of motion, or feeling more at peace and comfortable with your body, can often help you stay motivated. The progress journal techniques in this book are designed to assist you in monitoring these achievements and to give you tangible proof of your development. Additionally, this book's real-life success stories serve as a reminder that change is both possible and attainable.

Keep in mind that your path is distinct, and evaluating yourself against others may detract from the joy of your achievements. Focus on your goals, your route, and what's best for your mental and physical well-being. In this process, patience and self-compassion are just as important as commitment and discipline.

As you wrap up this book, keep in mind that chair yoga is a lifelong practice that will help you for years to come, not just a short-term weight loss solution. The mobility, strength, and flexibility you've acquired via chair yoga will enhance your quality of life and enable you to maintain your independence, vitality, and level of activity as you age.

Chair yoga offers more long-term advantages than just physical ones. It fosters spiritual connection, emotional stability, and mental clarity—all of which are necessary for a happy and healthy life. Chair yoga is an investment in your long-term health, regardless of whether you do it to lose weight, improve your mobility, or just feel more connected to your body.

You now possess the resources necessary to advance your career. Be consistent, pay attention to your body, and practice yoga and eating in a thoughtful, balanced manner. Your journey continues with every breath, stance, and deliberate meal; it doesn't end here.

Ultimately, there is more to this masterpiece than weight loss. It involves creating a way of living that supports mental, emotional, and physical wellness. Whether on the mat or in your daily life, every action you take moves you closer to becoming a stronger, healthier version of yourself.